AUTO-IMMUNITY AND AUTO-IMMUNE DISEASE

AUTO-IMMUNITY AND AUTO-IMMUNE DISEASE

A survey for physician or biologist

SIR MACFARLANE BURNET

MTP
MEDICAL AND TECHNICAL
PUBLISHING CO LTD
1972

Published by
MTP
MEDICAL AND TECHNICAL
PUBLISHING CO LTD
PO Box 55, St. Leonard's House
St. Leonard's Gate
Lancaster, Lancs.

ISBN 978-94-011-8097-9 ISBN 978-94-011-8095-5 (eBook)
DOI 10.1007/978-94-011-8095-5

First published 1972

The Garden City Press Limited
Letchworth, Hertfordshire
SG6 1JS

Contents

PREFACE vii

1 INTRODUCTION 1

2 THE STOCHASTIC APPROACH TO DISEASE 9

3 MODERN IMMUNOLOGICAL THEORY 33

4 TOLERANCE AND PARALYSIS 59

5 PHARMACOLOGICAL ASPECTS OF IMMUNE RESPONSES 73

6 INFECTION AND AUTO-IMMUNITY 87

7 AUTO-IMMUNE RESPONSES IN NORMAL ANIMALS 97

8 THE NEW ZEALAND MICE 109

9 DISEASES PRIMARILY INVOLVING BLOOD CELLS 121

10 GENERALIZED AUTO-IMMUNE DISEASES 131

11 LOCALIZED AUTO-IMMUNE DISEASES 153

12 PATHOGENESIS OF AUTO-IMMUNE DISEASE 173

13 POTENTIALITIES AND LIMITATIONS OF THERAPY 191

14 THE SIGNIFICANCE OF AUTO-IMMUNITY FOR AGEING 201

15 A PROGRAMME FOR THE FUTURE 213

ABBREVIATIONS 223

GLOSSARY 225

REFERENCES 229

INDEX 237

Preface

In 1957 or thereabouts I became impressed with how immunity could be looked at as a process of Darwinian selection amongst the circulating lymphoid cells of the body. The clonal selection theory which grew out of this has been generally accepted in principle by immunologists, but I do not feel that its full implications in relation to pathology have yet been widely realized. In a previous book, *Immunological Surveillance*, I have tried to apply the approach to cancer immunity. This is a basically similar attempt to look at auto-immune disease from the same Darwinian point of view.

Anyone who attempts to produce acceptable general statements about complex biological and clinical phenomena must have a certain sense of guilt. No biological phenomenon can ever be completely, or even adequately, described. There can, at best, only be a progressive improvement in the acceptability, the intellectual elegance, or the practical usefulness of the working generalizations that can be produced. Any attempt to write at this interpretative level can easily be brushed aside as superficial, unnecessary, and liable to be proved wrong or irrelevant by new developments. It is anathema to many good professional scientists and their objections are real enough.

Yet one can still ask whether there is any human significance in what we are doing if it does not help to provide, for those who want it, the best understanding of some corner of the universe in terms intelligible to the non-specialist and not currently at variance with the scientific record. This is not a book for the professional immuno-pathologist, but I hope it will be useful for anyone with a real peripheral interest in auto-immune phenomena to see its problems a little more clearly.

F. M. Burnet

AUTO-IMMUNITY AND AUTO-IMMUNE DISEASE

CHAPTER 1

Introduction

When an academic scientist retires he loses his salary and, unless he is very lucky, his secretary. Many other things that seemed important vanish, but there can be compensation in a new freedom. In a senior scientific post one's overriding concern is to try to ensure a satisfying career for the younger people who have come into research under one's aegis. It will do them harm if their sponsor is not well regarded by his senior contemporaries. In particular he must be seen to conform to the rules. There are rules about research which are vital to its integrity and which must never be broken; but there are others which are mere conventions. One is that the only legitimate activity for a scientist must be firmly centred on experimental work under his own control and in part at least done with his own hands. Another is expressed in Medawar's epigram that science is the art of the soluble: that it is only justifiable to ask questions in such a form that at least in principle they can be solved by acceptable experimental methods. As a working scientist I accepted them all as necessary and socially expedient just as I knew that it was wise to keep doubts about the human relevance of much good scientific work to myself. With retirement I have felt free to question them.

In particular I have relished the opportunity to try to see the outline of some of the woods in which I have spent my life examining twigs, branches, or even sometimes a whole tree. I am not self-disciplined enough to eschew the fascination of trying to correlate phenomena in terms of general concepts. The wider they are the more satisfying they feel. My justification, or rationalization, for applying this attitude to classes of phenomena which are admittedly too complex or too ill-defined to be ripe for generalization can be stated under three heads:

1. Any clearly stated hypothesis can stimulate good new experimental work to disprove, modify or confirm, and extend the theory in

question. I can claim with the support of a number of other immunologists that my (1957) clonal selection theory of immunity acted significantly as a catalyst to immunological research in the next decade.

2. Any generalization that covers a wide range of phenomena, even if its validity subsequently proves to be merely provisional and contemporary, can serve as an important aid to the practical man (usually a physician in my context) when he has to make an individual decision on what is always inadequate information. If someone generalizes that an 'auto-immune disease' has the basic quality of a conditioned malignancy due to one or a small number of mutant clones analogous to those of a lymphoma, the clinician may feel, for instance, that he is justified in testing cyclophosphamide or methotrexate as therapeutic agents.

3. Whenever an important new generalization emerges in one field of science, it is usually possible to see that a new need has risen to look at all the adjacent scientific areas in the light of the new concept. Every advance in organic chemistry (e.g. the use of nuclear magnetic resonance in resolving molecular structure) is soon applied to biochemical matters. In somewhat similar fashion any new enlightenment in theoretical immunology, cytology, or virology may have a bearing on the understanding of auto-immune disease. As long as science advances every major theme will need to be restated continually in the light of relevant advances in other fields.

As of 1971 every pathologist and every academically minded physician is aware that a steadily growing number of subacute or chronic diseases are being spoken of as auto-immune, i.e. resulting from misdirected immune responses against tissues or cells in the body. Not everyone believes that by calling a disease auto-immune or auto-allergic anything useful has been accomplished, and this attitude is reflected with various qualifications in most current medical and pathological writing.

In looking over immunological texts published since 1965 I can find no satisfactory general treatment of auto-immune disease based on modern immunological concepts. In many there is a hardly changed attitude that immunity means antibody and that antibody is constructed to a pattern appropriate to deal with antigen. The commonest suggestion is that, under the influence of drug or virus, cell antigens may be changed or previously segregated ones uncovered. The resulting immune response is responsible for the disease. The simple objection to this is that normal people suffer all types of infections, every variety of trauma, and are given many drugs. At least 99 per cent do not develop diagnosable auto-immune disease. To do so is always rare and most often there is no clear preceding cause or trigger. *A-priori* individual factors, presumably genetic and somatic genetic, would seem the most reasonable explanation for the rarity and individuality of cases of auto-immune disease.

There is a more deep-seated objection to any theoretical approach involving conceptions of somatic mutation or any similar processes. Many physicians and clinical scientists accept with varying degrees of explicitness that no disease condition can be understood other than as a result of some defined or definable impact of the environment on the body. They prefer to look for a slow virus, chronic poisoning by an industrial chemical or psychosocial trauma, rather than accept genetic or somatic-genetic processes, including auto-immune disease, as a valid interpretation of someone's illness. This I believe is an untenable position. There are important immunological anomalies in many disease conditions and in some the auto-immune character is almost self-evident.

My experience in writing at the theoretical level on immunological topics has been to find that most reviewers felt that speculation should stay much closer to the current state of experimental work, and that the only virtue of wider generalization was to suggest new experiments or new approaches to clinical management. I could claim, in extenuation, that the concepts introduced with the phrases 'clonal selection' and 'immunological surveillance' have been accepted as useful by immunologists and that the second is having a significant practical impact on the understanding of the appearance of malignant tumours in patients under immunosuppressive drug regimes. So, in attempting a book of similar type on auto-immune disease, I shall be concerned essentially in elaborating the idea of forbidden clones that from the first development of the clonal selection concept seemed to derive automatically from it. I still believe that, despite my failure to convince most immunologists of the usefulness of the approach, all new work on auto-immune disease is compatible with the idea and is progressively strengthening it.

The basic approach

Perhaps the two diseases which are most widely acceptable as auto-immune are acquired haemolytic anaemia (warm type) and Hashimoto's disease of the thyroid. Both, however, are still officially diseases of unknown etiology. About ten years ago the mouse strain NZB was shown to develop a reasonably accurate model of auto-immune haemolytic anaemia, and an F1 hybrid with another strain, NZW, derived from the same mixed stock showed regular development of lethal kidney lesions. It seemed that here was the material to establish the nature of auto-immune disease once and for all. After a dozen years of work in many laboratories there is still no interpretation that has been found generally acceptable. Even the self-evident genetic character of the disease has been called into doubt: it could be a vertically transmitted slow virus disease.

The objective in writing this book was to present as far as possible a consistent interpretation of both clinical and experimental phenomena of auto-immunity in terms of the clonal selection approach. To a considerable degree the first development of that approach in 1957 sprang from consideration of a case of macroglobulinaemia (proliferation of primitive lymphoid cells with production of excess immunoglobulin M) in whose blood Gajdusek and Mackay found a high titre of antibody reacting with human tissue extracts. Ever since then auto-immune disease has been a major interest. Much more is now known about the field, but the advances have not been revolutionary ones. My own approach is still expressed as a logical and lineal development of the forbidden clone concept formed within the framework of clonal selection theory in its first extended statement (Burnet, 1959). Like every conceivable interpretation it must constantly be updated and correlated with developments of other aspects of biology, in particular in the fields of general immunology and oncology. The hypothesis in its most generalized form will be as follows:

1. It is necessary for survival that neither immunocytes nor antibodies should exist in the body which are reactive to more than a minimal degree with any accessible body component.

2. Since immune pattern is generated by a random process a mechanism must exist by which any 'self-reactive' cells which may emerge can be eliminated or functionally inhibited. More than one mechanism may be needed to establish and maintain this intrinsic immunological tolerance toward self components.

3. There are many genetically determined anomalies in the functioning of the immune system ranging from agammaglobulinaemia, where the

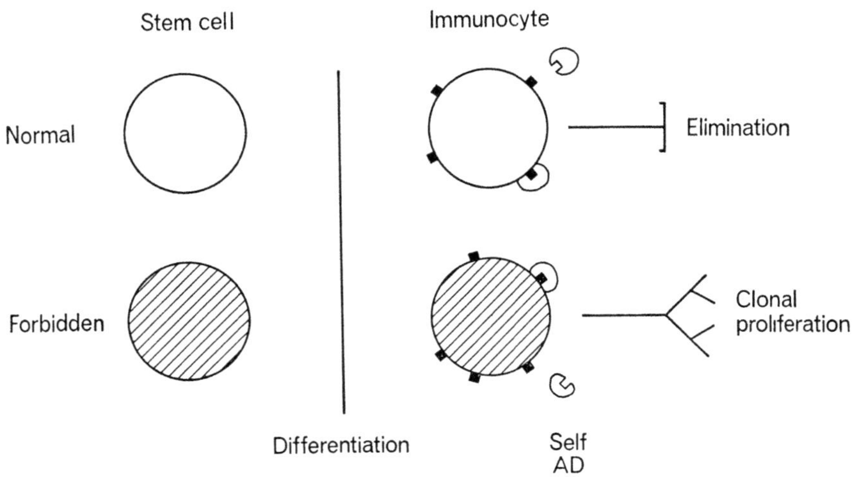

FIG. 1. The essence of the forbidden clone concept. A stem cell on differentiation becomes an immunocyte carrying a specific pattern of antibody-like receptors. If accessible antigenic determinants (AD) are present soon after differentiation any normal immunocyte capable of reacting with them will be eliminated. If, however, the stem line has undergone at some point a somatic mutation, increasing resistance (shaded), the differentiated immunocyte can, on specific stimulation, initiate a forbidden clone.

patient has no capacity to liberate antibody into the blood, to minor degrees of susceptibility to allergic reactions. Genetic susceptibility to develop auto-immune disease undoubtedly exists. Its basis has not been elucidated at either the genetic or the molecular level, but it is reasonable to suggest that it functions by shifting the 'point of decision' determining whether an immunocyte reacting with its corresponding determinant will be stimulated to proliferation and functional activity or will be destroyed or functionally inhibited.

4. Changes due to somatic mutation or to physiological or pharmacological factors may render a newly differentiated immunocyte (the antigen-reactive cell of most investigators) insusceptible to elimination or inhibition by the 'censorship' mechanism concerned. As in virtually every statement one can make in an immunological context, the word 'insusceptible' is not an absolute but simply refers to a range of susceptibility below the level, determined by genetic factors, of the normal newly differentiated immunocyte.

5. When, by somatic mutation, an immunocyte line develops which (*a*) has an undue resistance to elimination by antigenic contact and (*b*) reacts specifically with an accessible body component functioning

as antigenic determinant, it is potentially capable of initiating a forbidden clone of directly or indirectly pathogenic cells. As such they will have all the essential characteristics of a conditioned malignancy.

6. In all probability the clinical manifestations of auto-immune disease are due (*a*) to aggressive T-immunocytes (see p. 51 ff.) producing damage to target cells, (*b*) to the deposition of antigen-antibody complexes in the kidney or elsewhere, and (*c*) to a directly damaging action of antibody, but probably only when the auto-antigen is present in the circulating blood either on cells or as a soluble component.

7. The accessibility, amount, and physical character of the (auto-)antigen plays an essential part in determining both to what extent a potentially pathogenic clone is stimulated to proliferate and what opportunity it has to damage cells and tissues in the body.

It will be evident that this hypothesis of auto-immune disease is not one which can be stated bluntly and briefly in any such terms as 'a slow virus disease', 'the result of somatic mutation', 'due to antigen modification by virus or toxin', or 'a collagen disease'. To provide a reasoned argument for, and against, the theory as summarized, it seems necessary and logical to use the introductory chapters to discuss what seem to be relevant aspects of some more fundamental areas of biology.

The first can be spoken of broadly as the stochastic approach in biology which is concerned with the regularities that emerge from the occurrence of rare and random events with continuing consequences. In the field of mammalian pathology this must be concerned primarily with somatic mutation though there is a growing feeling that essentially similar processes are important in many of the normal functions of differentiation in the body. It is accepted by all that the generation of diversity of pattern in antibodies and immunocyte receptors has such an origin and it would be strange if similar principles did not apply elsewhere.

In so far as human disease (including auto-immune disease) is concerned, the most important observable consequence of any process involving somatic mutation is the age-specific incidence of the disease which results. For some diseases it may be possible to express the age incidence in terms of the total population at risk in each age-group. More often it is simpler to assess the percentage of all cases of disease that fall in each age-group. The criterion for selecting the significant date (and age) for each individual may be either by the onset of clinical disease, the appearance of a significant auto-antibody in the blood, or death from the disease. Burch's important work in this area will require sympathetic, if occasionally critical, discussion.

The second area is that of classical immunology, of which three particular fields bear most closely on auto-immunity. One concerns the apparently unique capacity of the immune system to produce by some type of randomized genetic process an immense diversity of immune patterns. Such immune patterns may be potentially useful, potentially dangerous, or simply irrelevant. This calls for means of getting rid of those that are potentially dangerous. Neglecting for the present some observational and logical difficulties, this is the basis of the important field of immunological tolerance. Auto-immune disease is, in the view to be adopted, the result of a failure to develop normal tolerance to some bodily component. The second field comprises what is probably the most significant development in recent immunology, the differentiation of the T and B immune systems concerned approximately with cell-mediated immunity and antibody production respectively. Both are deeply involved in auto-immune disease.

The third area for preliminary discussion is concerned with the principles of pharmacology in so far as they impinge on the production of cellular damage by immunological processes. Closely related and still far from being completely understood is the drug-like action of antigen (or antigenic determinant) on the specific receptors of the different varieties of immunocyte. It is perhaps significant of the possible breadth of this area that Boyden once put forward the view, admittedly only half seriously, that all inflammation is essentially an auto-immune reaction. It is quite difficult to find a formal disproof of such a thesis.

In undertaking a discussion of auto-immunity and auto-immune disease I have a fairly well-defined objective of the same type as I had in two previous books: *Self and Not Self*, a discussion of general immunological theory based on the clonal selection approach, and *Immunological Surveillance*, dealing with cancer immunity. The aim in all three has been to provide a general account which would be acceptable in outline to professional investigators in each field, but would be directed more to those interested in an attempt to look at clinical and pathological matters from a consistently biological angle. I do not think that it is only a reflection of my own interests to say that in the last two decades it is the biological disciplines concerned essentially with abnormality and infection, immunology, oncology, and virology which have contributed most to new understandings of the principles of biology. It is probably equally true to say that, for anyone seeking an understanding of the biology of man, the existence of cancer, auto-immune disease, and ageing are essential components of the whole human situation.

In any writing of this sort there are two related difficulties which in one, always unsatisfactory, way or another must be overcome. The relevant literature is far too large for anyone to read *in toto*, and reference to all the papers one has read and which seem relevant would hopelessly clog the sort of discussion required. The solution adopted is to state everything which appears to be broadly non-controversial without references unless there is special historical interest in quoting the circumstances of some discovery or new conception. Where a controversial situation has to be mentioned and either left unresolved or one of the alternatives accepted, a few key references will be given. It is inevitable that in the preliminary chapters a good deal of what was said in the earlier books will be paraphrased or summarized, but it will always be specifically slanted towards its relevance for the auto-immune phenomena with which we are concerned.

This is by no means a comprehensive clinical text and the discussion of clinical features is much more concerned to exemplify immunological principles than to offer help in diagnosis or treatment. However, most of the important auto-immune diseases of man are discussed at some length as well as a number of rarer conditions and some whose nature is still problematical. Considerable use will be made of experimental work both on normal animals and on genetically predisposed strains of mice, but nothing at all will be said about the examples of auto-immune disease that may be met with in veterinary practice.

CHAPTER 2

The stochastic approach to disease

In 1957–8 I was already deeply interested in what was coming to be called auto-immune disease and it became immediately obvious that if a clonal selection theory of immunity was to be accepted it must be applicable, with appropriate modifications, to pathological manifestations of immunity as well. The concept of the 'forbidden clone' emerged almost at once and I have seen no reason to withdraw the phrase or the idea since. It is a concept which can accept infinite elaboration to fit specific instances but yet remain basically very simple. In essence, a forbidden clone arises from a stem cell line in which two types of genetic individuality develop in the course of differentiation and somatic mutation. One is concerned with the nature of the 'immune receptor'. It must allow the immunologically reactive cell (immunocyte) to react specifically with some accessible component of the body acting as an antigenic determinant. The second is a genetic anomaly that makes the cell more resistant than normal to the processes which should result in the elimination of such autoreactive cells from the body. Instead, when conditions are appropriate, it is stimulated to proliferate to form a forbidden clone with potentially pathogenic effect.

In all essential respects a forbidden clone is equivalent to a clone of malignant cells. It is being stimulated to multiply by the constant availability of the corresponding antigen, although for reasons to be discussed later there is almost always some secondary control which prevents it developing into a full-blown malignant leukaemia or a near malignant macroglobulinaemia.

Much of what has been written about malignant disease is also applicable to auto-immune disease. In particular, the basic rule determining whether or not a somatic mutation is of any significance to the organism as a whole still holds. All mutations (i.e. all genetic changes which leave a cell still capable of mitosis) are rare, and random both in respect of time and of the informational content of the genome. There are sufficient cells in every functioning organ or system for functional abnormality of any sort in a *single* cell to be of no account. A functional abnormality only becomes significant when it endows the cell and its descendants with a capacity to build up an excessive clonal population.

Somatic mutation as exemplified in mammalian skin

It is almost conventional to label anyone postulating that such and such a phenomenon results from somatic mutation as an armchair theorist too lazy to analyse the phenomenon experimentally. There may be a faint basis for the accusation, for somatic mutation is a highly flexible concept which in the limit is almost equivalent to saying that by mutation a cell can lose or gain any qualities that the investigator cares to postulate. Yet exactly the same objection could be levelled at any discussion of the part played by point mutation, deletion, gene duplication, and other intragenomic processes in the germ line, in providing the raw material for evolution. Every observable quality of a living organism is accepted as being determined by, or at least deeply influenced by, genetic processes. At the somatic level everything suggests that very much the same processes can occur in the nucleus as take place in that of a germ-line cell. There is even some evidence that mutation can involve the same genes and take place with similar frequency at both levels.

It is quite impossible to understand auto-immune disease, or malignant disease, without making use of the concept of inheritable change in somatic cells.

In an attempt to clarify ideas on somatic mutation it seems expedient to discuss the one tissue of the body in which the effects are visible to any observer: the skin and its pigment cells (melanocytes).

Normal changes

There is almost a social obligation on the young in Australia to develop as extensive a sun-tan as convention and comfort will allow. The process is easier in some people than others but is possible to some extent in everyone who is not an albino. This can be regarded as an adaptive device involving all or most of the melanocytes and probably set in action by the mild inflammation of sunburn. This in turn is due to the shorter wavelengths of sunlight which impinge on the area exposed. As pigmentation increases, the effective wavelengths are absorbed before they can produce any inflammatory effect. The adaptive value of the response, which probably involves both an increase in the number of melanocytes and in their activity as melanin producers, is immediately evident.

Recently there has been some interesting discussion about the evolutionary processes that led to the appearance of the very lightly pigmented North European from the ancestral African hominids who must have been black- or brown-skinned. The suggestion is that the chief metabolic function of the skin is to convert inert sterols into calciferols with vitamin D activity. The near ultra-violet is necessary for this and in a high latitude both the amount reaching the skin and the amount of skin that can be exposed to light are reduced. So a minimum of shielding against the ultra-violet was desirable and the pigmentation of the skin grew progressively less. Obviously the melanocyte system must be capable of adaptation to the local environment at the level of the individual and of undergoing evolutionary changes dependent in the last analysis on germ-line mutations in the controlling genes.

In children and adults with genetically poor development of skin pigmentation—traditionally the small boy with red hair and thin, white skin—exposure of skin to sunlight results not in uniform tanning but in freckles. A freckle is a pigmented area resulting from the proliferation of a single melanocyte, originally located at the very centre of the circular freckle, to produce a clone of more than ordinarily active melanocytes. To the best of my knowledge no one has had the curiosity to apply modern scientific methods to find out the details of the freckling process, and its interpretation as resulting from somatic mutation is no more than a deduction from appearances. The facts are straightforward enough. Freckles are circular and enlarge periphally, their intensity of pigmentation is uniform over the whole circular area. In some children there are freckles of different intensities of pigmentation, as many as five different types being sometimes recognizable. The very dark brown freckles sometimes seen are smaller than the others and probably represent accumulations of more than one layer of melanocytes. Freckles develop preferentially in some areas of skin, but only in skin exposed to sunlight. They vary greatly in their subsequent history and probably most often fade into the general background of skin pigmentation.

I believe that a consideration of the basis of these appearances is directly relevant and rather helpful toward an understanding of what is involved in auto-immune disease. In both we adopt the hypothesis that somatic mutation is the basic process. In accounting for freckles we reach a number of conclusions that seem to be of general interest to biology and pathology. The first is that the mutation produced is such that its functional effect is very similar to what happens in all melanocytes of non-freckling individuals. It proliferates to some extent, produces on the average more melanin, and its descendants of the new clone move in such a fashion as to maintain a single layer with each melanocyte approximately the same distance from its neighbours. The mutation is induced by exposure to sunlight and, since ultra-violet light is a well-studied mutagenic agent in the laboratory, we assume that it is the shorter wavelengths that are responsible. Since the commonest thing to be observed as a result of mutation closely parallels an adaptive response, we must assume that what has been inheritably modified is that part of the somatic genome which determines the normal adaptive reaction. Some very interesting genetic problems (concerning the nature of 'phenocopies') arise here but are not relevant enough for discussion. We know that up to five pigmentary mutations can occur in the freckling process and it is a legitimate speculation that simultaneously a many times greater number of invisible and irrelevant mutations of other types occur in other cells of the melanocyte population. We can be certain that melanocytes move about, divide occasionally, and occasionally vanish. There is scope for competitive survival between clones and it is simplest to assume that non-proliferative mutations are either neutral or disadvantageous in the 'struggle for survival'. If such a mutant is in the area to be occupied by an active 'freckle' clone it will go to the wall.

The final point to be made is probably the most important of all: that the proliferating melanocytes are still under effective control. No freckle expands to cover more than a square centimetre and malignant melanoma never supervenes on a child's freckle. We do not know the nature of that control, but it impresses one as evidence that somatic mutation has been too important a factor in human and vertebrate evolution to be left without control. There is probably what in relation to auto-immune disease I called a 'fail-safe system' available for every important type of somatic

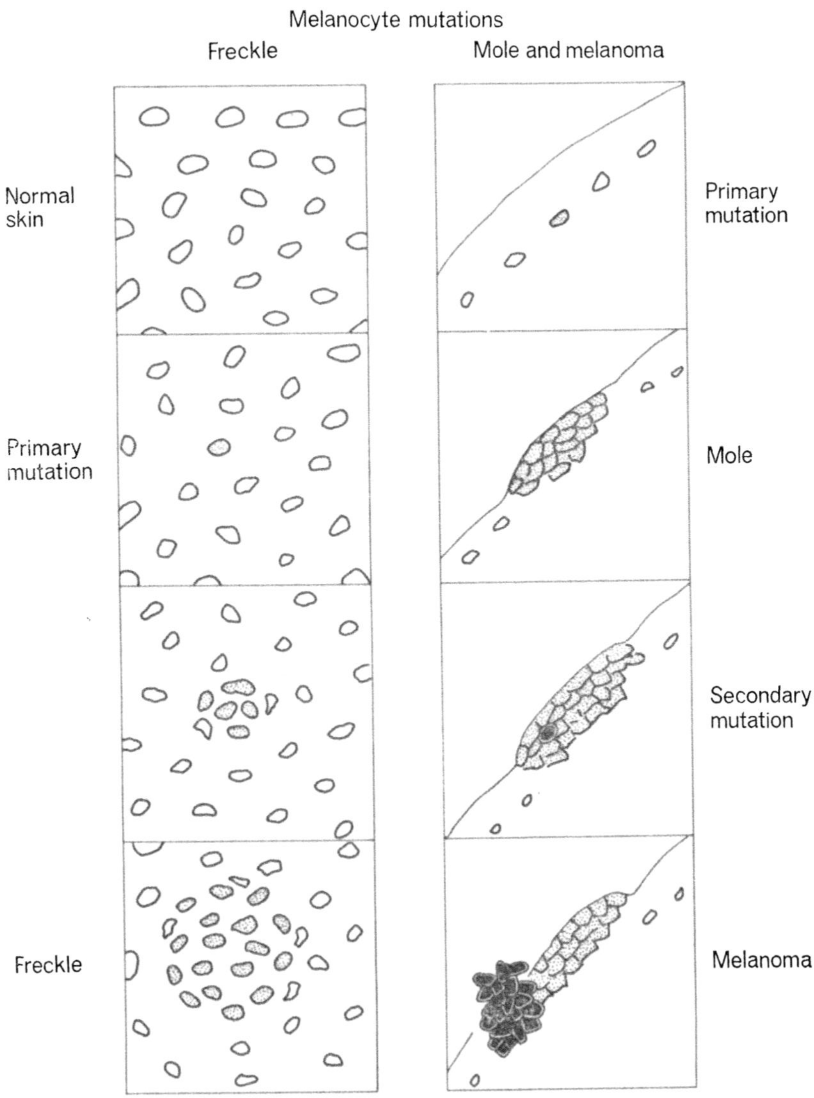

FIG. 2. Melanocyte mutations in human skin. Note the regular distribution of modified melanocytes in freckle and their irregular accumulation in mole and melanoma. Cells shown white are normal melanocytes, descendants of primary mutant stippled, secondary mutants black.

mutational anomaly, by which the clone can usually be inhibited or destroyed by two or more control systems. Only when all are overcome do we have the lethal somatic mutational diseases of cancer, systemic lupus erythematosus, and perhaps old age itself, but that is another story.

Moles and melanoma

There is, of course, a well-known cancer of the cells we are considering: malignant melanoma, still sometimes called melanotic sarcoma. Such tumours are very highly malignant as a rule, though occasionally, and more frequently than most other malignant tumours, they cure themselves spontaneously. Two other points of special interest in the present context are (*a*) that they arise usually from congenital moles and (*b*) that they are specially common in Europeans working in tropical or subtropical regions like Queensland.

As a preliminary to discussing malignant melanoma, something must be said about moles which are deep brown circular or oval patches often present at birth and composed of an accumulation of melanocytes not showing the normal orderly arrangement. Their natural history is variable; normally they enlarge somewhat with the child's growth and then stay virtually unaltered for life. Small ones sometimes disappear and careful examination of a child's skin will often show a small mole diminishing in size and surrounded by a narrow, pale areola unoccupied by melanocytes. The larger birthmarks are important because they represent mutations occurring for some unknown reason in melanoblasts (ancestral melanocytes) during foetal life. A particularly interesting one which I have seen demonstrated was an oval birthmark involving the upper eyelid and adjacent skin but with a small segment obviously of the same lesion on the lower eyelid. Here the main growth of the mutant clone of melanocytes had taken place when the skin over the orbit had not yet been cleaved to allow formation of the eyelids. The larger the birthmark the earlier was the initiating mutation. There is something to suggest that somatic mutation can occur at any stage of development from the first divisions of the fertilized egg onward. The evidence for this, however, comes from another source and will be mentioned later.

A mole, then, is a clonal accumulation of melanocytes whose most obvious abnormality is the loss of the normal habit of distributing themselves uniformly in the deeper layer of the skin epidermis. They are not responding to one of their cues for normal behaviour in relation to the rest of the tissue and in this sense can be regarded as on the road to malignancy. Trauma and prolonged exposure to strong sunlight can apparently sometimes induce a further mutation which can overcome the residual controls which had kept the mole quiescent for many years. This provides an opportunity to introduce the concept of sequential mutation. The chance of any given somatic mutation occurring in a given cell is always very rare. If its frequency is expressed as $1/n$, n will probably be of the order 10^5–10^8. The probability of the same cell undergoing two unrelated mutations will be $1/n' \times 1/n''$, which will usually be prohibitively small. There are, however, two ways in which sequential mutations can occur. If mutation results in a cell with such a proliferative advantage that in a reasonable period of time it has, say, 10^6 descendants all carrying the mutant characteristic, this is a population of cells in which mutation 2 can occur. If the joint effect of 1 and 2 is to produce malignant character in the cell, it will in due course give rise to a malignant clone. The example of malignant melanoma arising on an ordinary mole is a legitimate prototype of what has often been regarded as the standard way in which a malignant tumour arises.

The second way by which sequential mutation can be facilitated can also be exemplified in the pathology of moles. It is common observation that moles and birthmarks are much commoner in some children than others and that the tendency is sometimes inheritable. Here one must assume that the genetic anomaly, presumably arising by germ-line mutation in some ancestor, renders the genome abnormally susceptible to mutate in this particular direction under a stimulus that would be ineffective in a standard cell. The possibility that the same undue susceptibility can be induced by *somatic* mutation is not easy to test. It is supported, but whether relevantly or not is doubtful, by the almost regular phenomenon of 'progression' that is observed in experimentally transplantable tumours. The very process of successive transfer of a tumour from one individual to another of a more or less homozygous strain of animals is a continuing challenge for any mutants to proliferate with selective advantage. In fact there is rather regularly a progressive increase in malignant activity often associated with gross chromosomal abnormality and sometimes with capacity to grow in unrelated hosts of the same species.

Pigmentation in albinos

There is a further manifestation of somatic mutation as it affects human skin pigmentation which has its own special interest in a general context. Albinism is not uncommon in many dark-skinned races and I have some personal experience of its occurrence in the Trobriand Islands and northern New Guinea. It is a genetic condition due to a recessive gene which prevents one stage of the synthesis of melanin from tyrosine. Albino children are born with quite unpigmented skin, but as they age pigmented spots appear in the skin, some of which develop into larger areas. From limited observation there are considerable individual differences in the types of pigmented areas which are observed, and quite obviously there is a rich field here for biochemical and somatic genetic investigation. The main possibilities are that an effective reverse mutation to that responsible for the original germ-line mutation has taken place or that the primary enzymic block has been circumvented in some different fashion.

Most of those interested in the genetics of protein structure would regard a true reverse mutation, i.e. when the mutation A to B resulting from a single nucleotide change is directly reversed B to A, as almost vanishingly unlikely and prefer to explore the possibility that a variety of other changes in the gene and its derivative enzyme may re-establish more or less effective action of the enzyme. With modern microchemical methods it should be possible to obtain direct evidence of the processes concerned.

Fleece mosaics in sheep

This discussion of somatic mutation in relation to superficially visible abnormalities of the skin can be concluded by moving to another species, the sheep, and another skin product, the fleece. It is important as providing evidence that a somatic mutation can occur even in the earliest stages of segmentation of the fertilized egg. I have retold the story due to Fraser and Short (1958) several times in books and lectures, but it remains the best example of the phenomenon it illustrates.

It is well known to Australian sheep-breeders that lambs are occasionally born with some abnormality of the fleece. For obvious reasons they are culled as soon as the abnormality is recognized, unless a research organization is interested in the phenomenon. The Australian CSIRO (Commonwealth Scientific and Industrial Research Organization) was interested and had access by proxy to flocks totalling some 20 million sheep. With good co-operation by owners and managers Fraser and Short collected 22 sheep of merino and crossbred strains in which portion of the normally compact, closely crimped fleece was replaced by areas of long, almost uncrimped fibres. It is an abnormality easily visible when sheep are yarded for shearing and at least all the gross examples were probably obtained for examination. Even with the small numbers available for study there was a striking regularity in the inverse relationship between the size of the area occupied by the long mutant wool and the frequency of its occurrence. There was 1 sheep with 50 per cent of its skin area involved, 3 with 25 per cent, 5 with about 12 per cent, and the other 13 with smaller areas. The only obvious interpretation was that the long fleece represented the result of a mutation that could occur with equal frequency in any cell of any cell generation of early embryonic development. The animal with 50 per cent long wool was the only one in which the first segmentation division was involved. When four cells were present a mutation should only involve a quarter of the fleece but be twice as frequent and so on. The findings agree and there is no other simple interpretation. The hypothesis, which is Fraser's and Short's, cannot be regarded as proven, but I can see no alternative and it has several important implications that are probably relevant to the genetics of immunity and auto-immune disease.

In the first place a mutation in one of the cells from the primary division of the ovum must be present eventually in half the cells of the body, but there is no evidence of any resulting abnormality in such sheep other than the fleece-mosaic quality. A somatic mutation of highly specific character then can occur in a cell long before differentiation has begun. It is only in descendant cells differentiating in such a fashion that the specific quality can be phenotypically expressed that the mutant character is shown. The patches of long wool have a characteristic distribution in more or less lens-shaped areas running down from back to belly: a manifestation of the complex wanderings of stem cells after the time that they had been

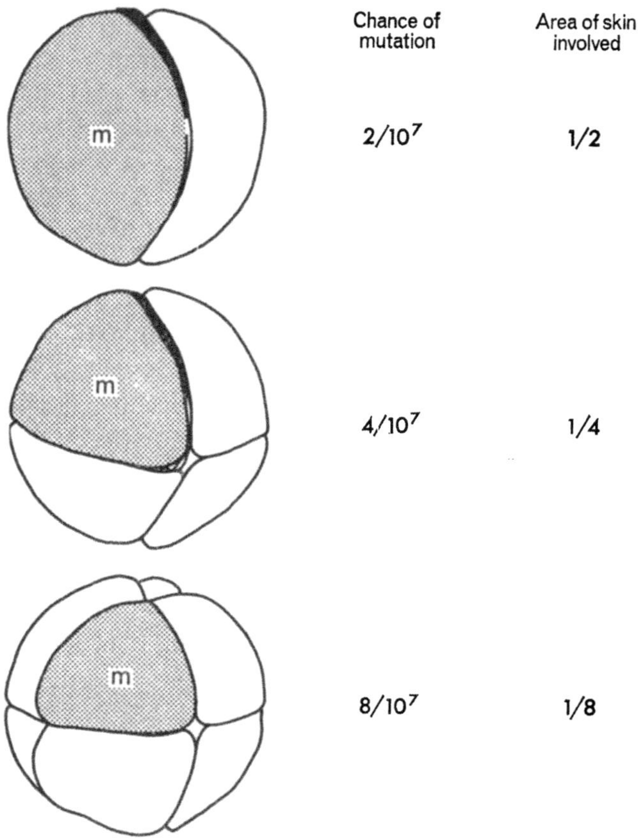

FIG. 3. The origin of fleece mosaics in sheep. The diagram is intended to illustrate the likelihood of somatic mutation during the earliest stages of embryonic development and the consequent area of skin involved. Mutations at later stages will be more frequent and the proportion of abnormal fleece smaller.

'chosen' by preliminary differentiation for a role in the skin. There are interesting analogies to these sheep in the 'composite' mice that can be produced by fusing early mouse embryos of different strains to form a single blastocyst and eventually a viable 'allophenic mouse' (Mintz). Where there are coat colour differences between the two component strains the composite mouse shows a rather similar arrangement of irregularly alternating stripes.

The age incidence of auto-immune disease

Since 1963 P. R. J. Burch has used my concept of the 'forbidden clone' to study the implications of the age and sex incidence of auto-immune and other chronic human diseases. I have been in fairly close touch with Burch throughout and although I have found it impossible to follow some of Burch and Burwell's biological theorizing I regard this work as of great importance for the understanding of auto-immune disease.

There is a large branch of mathematics concerned with the regularities of stochastic processes, i.e. processes by which events occurring wholly at random can, where large numbers of such events are considered together, be shown to have regularities susceptible to mathematical expression. The classical example is the regularity of radioactive decay with its standard 'half life' for each type of nuclear disintegration. Molecular movement and collision is wholly random as far as any individual molecule is concerned, but the gas laws and the equations governing diffusion in liquids are indicative of the regularities which emerge.

For many years there have been available in advanced countries detailed statistics of death. Increasingly we have available for every death as it occurs information as to sex, age at death, and the attending physician's assessment of primary and contributory causes of death. This provides the most accessible and in many ways the most important material for the study of stochastic regularities in human disease.

When we are concerned with a particular disease as such, irrespective of whether or not it terminates in death, the most desirable information is the age of onset of diagnosable disease. For such conditions as those we are concerned with this may be hard to specify at all exactly. An alternative that may be available is to take the cross-section of people of all ages and note how many of them at that particular time show evidence of past or continuing experience of any disease like rheumatoid arthritis that leaves a characteristic deformity. All such records need effort for their collection and the data must be examined very critically for a variety of errors and uncertainties. More or less satisfactory data obtained by one or other of these methods is available for most of the commoner auto-immune diseases. Those which seemed adequate for the purpose have been used by Burch for his mathematical analyses.

The simplest approach to Burch's work is probably to start with its application to the age incidence of the various forms of malignant disease as defined by age at death from cancer.

Malignant disease analogies

Cancer of accessible organs (skin, breast, uterus, tongue, testis) will nearly always be correctly diagnosed on death certificates. It was obvious that all such cancers are more frequent in old age and physicians with statistical and mathematical interests have many times studied the regularities of the age-specific incidence of death from the various types of cancer. If we deliberately neglect all second order effects, age-specific incidence curves for human cancers take the form of a straight line with a slope of four or five when the age-specific incidence and the ages are both plotted on a logarithmic scale. It is usual to use five- or ten-year intervals and express, for example, the age-specific incidence of lung cancer in men aged 40–44 years as the number of reported deaths per annum for every 100,000 men in that age-group alive at the beginning of the year or quinquennium concerned. A regularity of this sort calls for interpretation and many statisticians and epidemiologists have interested themselves in the problem. The simplest and perhaps most likely explanation is that the curve represents the effect of rare and random cellular changes occurring over a prolonged period of time and, once induced, persisting indefinitely in the cells concerned and their descendants. In less general terms the postulate is that a rare somatic mutation, which may occur at any time during the life of the organism, confers a proliferative advantage on that cell over similar but unmutated cells. Such cells may then suffer another or a sequence of mutations each of which raises the proliferative advantage until an eventual clone of cells has the quality of malignancy.

It is of special interest that, in mice particularly, a tendency to develop cancer, often of one particular type, may be an inherited characteristic. Sometimes it is necessary to express the susceptibility to cancer as making it more likely that an environmental agent will initiate a cancerous process. This may be an oncogenic virus in some mouse strains or the irritation of weed burrs on the skin of a strain of sheep in Australia. An even more clear-cut example of inheritance of an enhanced liability to malignant disease can be observed in man.

A not very uncommon tumour of the eye in children, retinoblastoma, has been known for many years to be, in part at least,

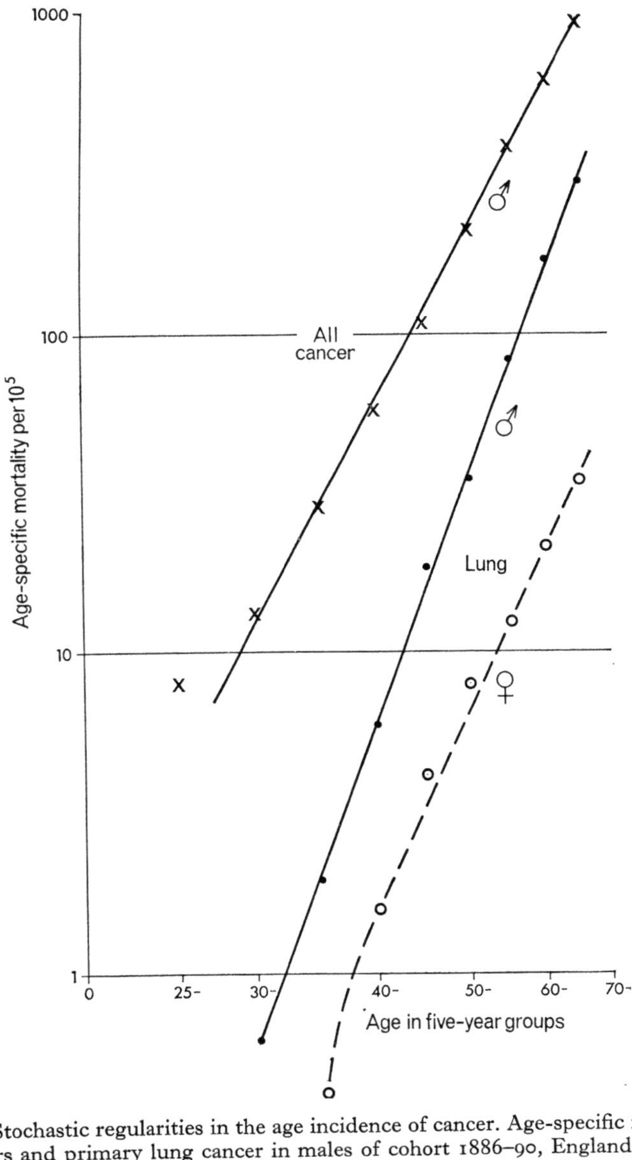

FIG. 4. Stochastic regularities in the age incidence of cancer. Age-specific incidence of all cancers and primary lung cancer in males of cohort 1886–90, England and Wales, and lung cancer in females of the same cohort. Age-specific mortality per 10^5 plotted against age in years, both scales being logarithmic.

inheritable as a dominant characteristic with incomplete penetrance and occasionally spontaneous recovery. It has now provided an example of the *same* mutation occurring either in a germ cell or a somatic cell. Knudson (1971), developing in part ideas from previous workers, has shown convincingly that retinoblastoma depends on two sequential mutations, the first of which can be either germinal or somatic, the second is necessarily somatic. His statistical calculations are based on the evidence that bilateral tumours are always inherited, while about 20 per cent of unilateral tumours are also inherited. The other 80 per cent (55·65 per cent of the total cases) are of the non-hereditary type. Other data concern the number of separate tumours and the age at diagnosis.

Retinoblastomas are derived from a cell, which gives rise to the ganglion cells amongst other types, and which progressively disappears during infancy. At birth there are approximately 2×10^6 cells at risk in each eye. The quantitative data are consistent with the tumour being initiated by two mutations, the first of which is dominant when it occurs at the germinal level. The rate of the second mutation (somatic) in carriers of the first is of the order of 2×10^{-7} per year. Knudson calculates a germinal mutation rate of about 5×10^{-6} per generation for the first mutation and the results are consistent with the somatic rate for this mutation being of the same order. As would be expected, the bilateral cases which must necessarily have a hereditary component appear earlier than the unilateral group, 80 per cent of which result from a sequence of two somatic mutations. The average time of recognition of the former is 15 months, while it is from 24 to 32 months in different series for the latter. More important than the average, however, is the distribution of cases according to age of onset. The shape of the appropriate curves fully supports the deduction of the essential equivalence of germinal and somatic mutation in this instance. It provides in fact an important support for the interpretation of some auto-immune phenomena on basically similar lines by Burch over the last eight or nine years.

Application to auto-immune disease

I had already suggested that a forbidden clone of auto-immune cells had a close formal resemblance to a conditioned neoplasm. Burch therefore began an analysis (by stochastic mathematical methods) of the age-specific incidence curves of a wide range of auto-immune

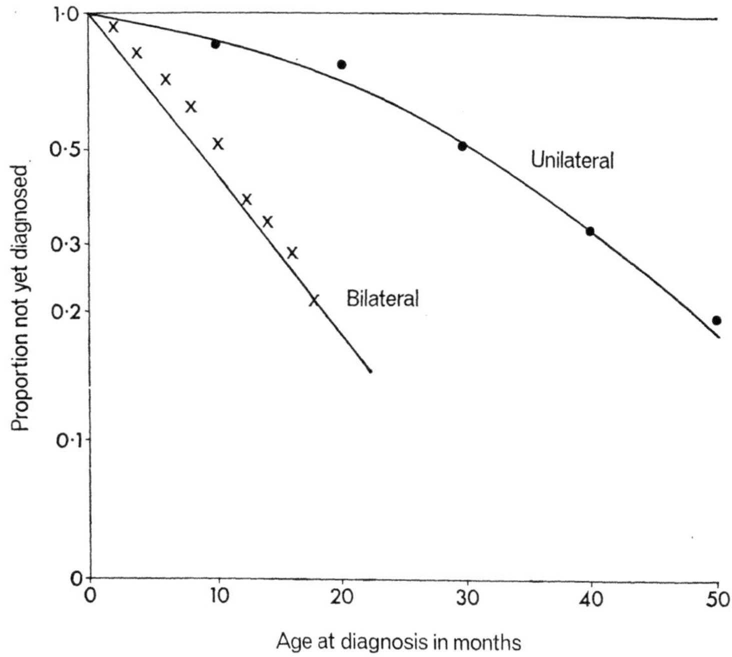

FIG. 5. Semilogarithmic curves of proportion of cases 'not yet diagnosed' by months for unilateral and bilateral cases of retinoblastoma. Redrawn from Knudson to show the earlier appearance of the bilateral disease and the approximate correspondence to one-hit (bilateral) and two-hit (unilateral) curves.

and degenerative diseases. His first paper was concerned with rheumatoid arthritis or, more specifically, with that aspect of it which can be defined as inflammatory polyarthritis. Since then he has applied a similar approach to virtually every subacute and chronic human malady not clearly infective in origin for which reasonably comprehensive data on age incidence are available. More will be said about Burch's approach to the whole range of arthritic conditions in a later section. Burch's results with auto-immune and 'probably auto-immune' conditions may be summed up in his own words as 'consistent with the following generalizations.

1. When predisposition to the disease is limited to one or more groups of people within the general population, the specificity of such groups is determined by genetic factors.

2. The initiation of the disease process is contingent upon the occurrence of one or a small number of random events. The random events are identified as somatic gene mutations. In analysing the age

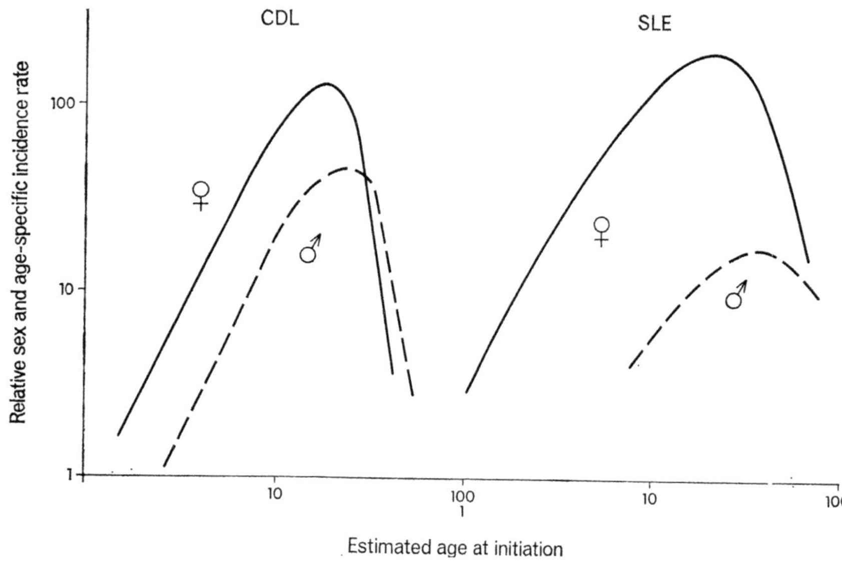

FIG. 6. Burch and Rowell's curves for chronic discoid lupus (CDL) and systemic lupus erythematosus (SLE) (redrawn). The relative sex and age-specific initiation rate plotted against the estimated age at initiation, both on logarithmic scales. The curves are drawn to give the best fit for an initiation rate proportional to $t^2 \exp(-kt^3/3)$. CDL = Burch and Rowell, *Lancet*, **ii** (1963), 509; SLE (U.S. data) = *Acta derm-venereol. (Stockholm)*. **50** (1970), 293–301.

incidence the following subsidiary assumptions about the somatic mutations are used:

a. The average rate of mutation is constant from around birth through to growth and maturity;

b. Rate is the same in all predisposed individuals and is independent of environment.

3. An interval elapses between the last random initiating event and the first onset of symptoms and signs. This may extend to as much as 25–30 years.'

As examples at this stage we can use the findings for systemic lupus erythematosus (SLE) and chronic discoid lupus (CDL). The age incidence curves plotted logarithmically on both axes are shown. The great excess (about eightfold) of females with SLE is ascribed to three mutant (germ-line) genes on the X chromosome; one only is needed in CDL. From the shape of the age-specific incidence rate curves it is deduced that for SLE three somatic mutations involving the X chromosome must occur, giving rise to three pathogenic cell clones. For

CDL one somatic mutation in an X chromosome and two autosomal ones are postulated. The curves for both SLE and CDL are fitted to the equation

$$\frac{dN}{dt} \propto t^2 \exp\left(\frac{-kt^3}{3}\right)$$

Other statisticians and geneticists have suggested that Burch may be over-elaborating his interpretations. The precise nomination in biological terms of the rare and random events indicated by the mathematics will always be difficult. There have been at least three different interpretations at the cellular level for the simple straight line shown by several types of cancer when the age incidence is plotted in this log–log fashion. While fully conscious that I am no mathematician, I should prefer, as a biologist, not to go much beyond Burch's three basic generalizations noted above.

It may, for instance, be quite sufficient, in discussing the SLE curve, simply to make the three points:

1. There is good evidence for genetic mutant genes being required.
2. A complex and variable constellation of antibodies and almost certainly of T-auto-immunocytes must have arisen by somatic mutation on some equivalent process.
3. A latent period is needed before a clone can increase to the numbers needed for a pathogenic effect.

On general grounds one would feel that a *sine qua non* for any detailed stochastic analysis was a clearly definable nosological entity with universally accepted criteria for diagnosis. This is far from being the case for SLE or indeed for any of the more extensively studied auto-immune conditions. The essence of SLE is the heterogeneity and variability of signs and symptoms and the wide range of overlap with auto-immune conditions which must be placed in some other category.

Another, but generally less important, difficulty is that of giving a definite date (and hence age) of onset of significant symptoms. Burch has suggested, apropos of rheumatoid arthritis, that if one could extract certain specific aspects of the disease picture as being diagnostic of clone *A*, others of clones *B*, *C*, etc., then tabulation of the ages of onset of each sign might allow a clearer picture, and again, assuming accurate reporting of the facts, one can concur.

Relation to growth and maintenance of cells

Burch's work on the stochastic analysis of the age incidence of auto-immune and degenerative disease is of the highest significance but hardly justifies the theoretical superstructure that he and Burwell have erected upon it. This assumes that growth and maintenance of normal cellular relationships is mediated by a central mechanism, which can sense the size of the growing target tissue and respond appropriately to influence the mitotic rate: negative feedback control, in other words. If organ *A* sends too many 'messages' into the centre, this must release mitosis inhibitors specific for that organ or tissue. The mitosis inhibitors, in their view, are 'mitotic control proteins', which may exist in a form carried by circulating lymphocytes or as a soluble plasma protein, probably an $\alpha 2$ globulin. It is assumed that there may be as many as 10^8 different patterns of tissue specificity amongst the cell surface antigens and mitotic control proteins.

A similar but less highly elaborated approach dealing with the same general problems of structural homoeostasis is Bullough's chalone theory. Using Bullough's own brief summary: 'The rate of production of new cells is determined from moment to moment by a negative feed-back system . . . the cells synthesize a tissue-specific antimitotic messenger molecule called a chalone which limits the rate of cell production' (Bullough, 1971). The antimitotic power is strengthened by two stress hormones (adrenaline and a gluco-corticoid hormone). No cellular antimitotic messengers are postulated and the number of specific types of chalone is not discussed.

There is at present no accepted theoretical formulation of the process of morphogenesis or of homoeostatic control of adult structure essentially because of the lack of any relevant experimental approach. If a satisfactory theory is eventually developed it will undoubtedly need to be considered in relation to auto-immunity, degenerative disease, and ageing, but for the present one must remain wholly sceptical.

In the absence of a more refined methodology virtually all current concepts of central control of regeneration (and by implication of morphogenesis and morphological homoeostasis) derive from experiments on the rat liver. The usual objective of the experiments is to show that surgical removal of 50 per cent or more of the normal liver tissue has an effect on liver cell mitosis which is demonstrable not only in the remaining portion of the liver but also on any other liver tissue so placed as to be perfused by the same circulating blood. If the experimental rat *A* has well-established autologous liver grafts elsewhere in the body or if the rat *A* is parabiosed with a syngeneic 'indicator' rat *B*, then removal of two-thirds of the liver from *A* is soon followed by a burst of mitosis in the remaining liver tissue and in the grafts or the liver of parabiont *B*. This effect must be mediated by some humoral mechanism, but none of those suggested seems particularly convincing. One suggestion is that each cell liberates a specific chalone which is mitosis-inhibitory when it returns to the cell via the blood stream. Removal of half the liver diminishes the concentration in the blood and the intrinsic mitotic potential of the cells is released. An alternative suggestion is that an abnormally low concentration of specific tissue molecules in the blood is recognized at some central control station and a compensatory release of mitosis-stimulating cells or substances takes place. This is a simplified form of the hypothesis favoured by Burch and Burwell. A third and more promising suggestion comes from the indication that the mitogenic stimulus for the liver comes via the portal blood (Fisher *et al.*, 1971). It seems a far more reasonable thought that part of the stimulus for a mutilated organ to regenerate springs from a 'recognition' that its function is inadequate. The liver has many functions, most of them concerned with the uptake and metabolic disposition of substances reaching it from the portal system. In the normal condition the number of cells handling metabolite *A* will be adequate to reduce the concentration of *A* in the liver-sinus blood to a standard level. Any progressive rise in that level will be expected, first, to raise the metabolic activity in the cells dealing with *A*, and, if it continues, to induce a mitotic response that will make more functional cells available. Following gross removal of liver tissue, all types of metabolic function will be more or less inadequate for normal requirements and a widespread burst of mitosis will be induced. This seems to provide the most reasonable interpretation of the experimental findings. Similar interpretations at a functional level could easily be developed for other organs.

It is simplest, therefore, to take the point of view that the essential process in morphogenesis is contact interaction between cells governed by information in the differentiated somatic cell genome. In no serious sense has morphogenesis anything to do with auto-immune disease.

As Burch has himself pointed out: 'This stochastic interpretation of the initiating process conformed perfectly with Burnet's (1959) forbidden clone theory of auto-immunity which I was engaged in testing. Although it was interesting and even important to discover that auto-immune diseases are probably initiated by only a few random events, it was far from puzzling because it verified Burnet's prediction.' I am highly appreciative of Burch's work and I believe that his application of a stochastic approach represents the most powerful confirmation of a line of biological thought that has been a guiding principle of mine since the mid 1950s. I shall use his results extensively with only an occasional use of *as if* when I feel that the deduction from a log–log plot of clinical data and a fitted curve is just a little too detailed.

Population dynamics of circulating body cells

Much of immunology and many aspects of pathology are concerned basically with the population genetics and dynamics of the circulating cells of the body. The approach must be essentially similar to the ecological and evolutionary study of individuals and species of nature. Population genetics is the basis of modern evolutionary theory and is concerned primarily with the factors, genetic and environmental, which are responsible for the numbers and distribution of genotypes of the species under study. The environment is important largely by its influence on the selective survival of various phenotypes. The population genetics of any natural species reproducing sexually is always greatly complicated by the heterozygosity of every individual and the difficulties of deducing genotype from the observable phenotypic characters.

In dealing with what happens to cell populations within an individual mammal we are (or may be) concerned with a simpler situation. There seems to be no valid evidence for assuming that somatic cell hybridization, recombination of genetic material or transfer of genetic material from one somatic cell to another plays any part in the physiological functioning of any higher vertebrate. An immense variety of such interactions are known to occur in bacteria, and laboratory analogues with mammalian cells in culture have been widely described. Genetic information of viral origin can under appropriate conditions be implanted in vertebrate cells and transform them to malignancy. A good case can also be made for transfer by oncogenic virus of fragments of genetic information from one mammalian cell to another, in a fashion analogous to transduction in bacteria. Elaborate and highly artificial circumstances are required for the demonstration of such phenomena in the laboratory and I know of no demonstration that any physiological transfer of genetic information between somatic cells occurs in vertebrates. It has often been invoked to explain laboratory artifacts in the fields of immunology and oncology, but none of these interpretations has yet been accepted by more than a handful of investigators with some commitment to the doctrine. Transfer of information *may* occur *in vivo*, but the only conceivable way in which it could be manifest would be in regard to the properties of a tumour arising from the recipient cell. Since there is general agreement, with some substantial if very incomplete experimental backing, that every somatic cell contains in its genome all the information present in every other cell in the body, it would be formally impossible to prove transfer of information of physiological significance. Any serious discussion of the population dynamics of lymphocytes and other circulating body cells must be based on the postulates that interaction between somatic cells is either due to cell to cell contact involving receptors and effectors of the cell surface or mediated by soluble substances liberated into the local micro-environment or the circulation and affecting receptors on appropriate cells. In other words, we are concerned only with successive stages of differentiation, clonal proliferation, distribution of cells as between free circulation and location in solid tissues, and the various ways in which cells die or are released into the external environment.

Development and function of lymphocytes

It has proved quite extraordinarily difficult to sort out the origin and fate of the cell which by common consent is the most important type concerned with immunological reactions, the small lymphocyte. A survey of these difficulties and the methods used to overcome them is a useful introduction to what is known in regard to the population dynamics of any type of circulating cell.

The first point to be stressed about the small lymphocyte is its intrinsic anonymity. It has a standard nucleus containing, by accepted teaching, all the potential information in any other cell of the body but with virtually none of it phenotypically expressed. The cytoplasm, within which the functional activity of most differentiated cells is expressed, is meagre in the small lymphocyte and, apart from a sparse scattering of the organelles characteristic of all cells, contains nothing of note either under the optical microscope or by electron microscopy. For many years it was orthodox teaching that the small lymphocyte was an end cell which might persist in the body for long periods, but eventually disappeared by autolysis or by release on to an environmental surface such as the intestinal mucosa. Only in 1960 did it become clear that a relatively large proportion of circulating small lymphocytes could be stimulated by kidney bean extract phytohaemagglutinin (PHA), to enlarge, undergo mitosis, and multiply for several generations in an appropriate medium. This soon became the commonest method of obtaining dividing human cells in metaphase for karyotyping. A year or two earlier Gowans had shown that small lymphocytes from the thoracic duct of rat *A*, when injected into F1 hybrids *A/B*, provoked a graft versus host reaction that was often fatal. If the *A* cells were appropriately labelled with amino acid carrying a suitable radio-isotope, they lodged largely in spleen and lymph nodes. Twenty-four hours later the labelled cells had taken on the form of large pyronophil cells with active nucleoli. This strongly suggested that the foreign histocompatibility antigen in the *A/B* hybrid had stimulated the lymphocytes to enlarge and undergo mitosis.

The broad point of view to be adopted can be visualized from this experiment of Gowans. The lymphocyte is basically a carrier of information which will be of value in certain emergency situations. As will emerge when we consider immunological functions more closely, that information may be of many different types, but for the present this diversity may be neglected and we can say that the lymphocyte is capable of two roughly alternative activities. On specific stimulation the potential information is expressed by functional and morphological changes involving the cytoplasm. The cell may be transformed into a lymphoblast from which a fresh clone of lymphocyte derives or into a plasmablast from which a clone of cells producing one or other type of immunoglobulin will arise. Multiplication of a single cell to produce a clone requires, of course, a supply of all the chemical building blocks and the energy to make, say, a hundred cells to the pattern of one. The initial cell of the clone can be said to supply all the information needed, but the substance must come from elsewhere. This introduces what appears to be the second, so-called trophic, function of the lymphocyte, to serve as a mobile store of material which can, as it were, be cannibalized at random for the building of the currently needed type. Lymphocytes are readily damaged, for example, by cortisol, and autolyse easily. If in a collection of a thousand lymphocytes each with its own specific potentiality there is one cell only of the type needed and a hundred of them are wanted as soon as possible, the logical

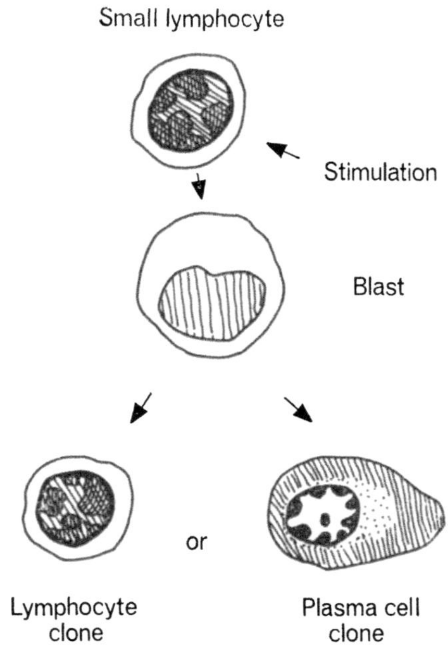

FIG. 7. Morphological potentialities of the small lymphocyte.

approach is obvious. A hundred of the lymphocytes must be autolysed at random and the resulting chemical building blocks made available for the development of the needed clone. This is, of course, an absurdly simplified model, but in essence it probably offers a legitimate way of looking at the double function of the lymphocyte.

Much experimentation in cellular immunology is designed to find the source of lymphocytes which at some later stage develop into a morphologically or functionally definable cell type. In general, the approach is to administer an appropriate label to a donor animal and at the desired period transfer a cell population from circulating blood, thymus, bone marrow, etc., to a syngeneic animal. The distribution of labelled cells in the recipient and any morphological changes that had taken place provided the basis for functional deductions.

Detailed applications of this technique call for much ingenuity but also demand caution in interpreting the results. One virtually never obtains a 95–100 per cent concordance in favour of one interpretation and the results usually can only be taken as predominantly favouring one view but never quite eliminating alternatives. Without attempting to provide experimental justification for the statements, the following probably represents the greatest common measure of agreement by those who have worked in this general field.

From an early stage of embryonic development in bird or mammal accumulations of non-specialized cells can be recognized as being the site of origin of the red cells and granulocytes of the blood as well as a variety of indeterminate mononuclear forms including lymphocyte-like cells. These haematopoietic areas are successively in the yolk sac area, in liver and spleen, and, after birth, in the bone marrow. It is assumed that there is a continuing proliferation of stem cells which morphologically are not distinguishable from large or medium lymphocytes. A basic stock of stem cells is always retained in the haematopoietic region, but from a certain stage there is a steady liberation of cells for specialized differentiation. It is unknown where and when a stem cell is irreversibly 'predestined' to give rise to erythrocyte, granulocyte, or lymphocyte, and from our point of view it is probably unimportant.

The natural history of the lymphocyte can be said to begin when stem cells enter the epithelial prototype of the thymus, and proliferate to form the mass of thymocytes that eventually makes up the cortex. Morphologically these cells are lymphocytes. In the chicken a similar process takes place in the bursa of Fabricius, where again lymphocyte-like cells develop which are presumed to be ancestral to plasma cells. It is uncertain whether there is any mammalian analogue to the bursa. A widely held opinion is that there are several regions of gut-associated lymphoid tissue (GALT), including appendix, tonsil, and Peyer's patches, which might have an equivalent function.

It would be in accord with most findings to assume that until a stem cell lodges in one of these two sites it has no capacity to react with antigen but that as it proliferates in the epithelial environment it differentiates to an immunocyte. This can be defined as a cell producing antibody/immunoglobulin which can function as a surface receptor and in some forms is synthesized and liberated in quantity. The term antigen-reactive cell (ARC) is commonly used by investigators in this field to distinguish the earliest forms of immunocyte.

When we speak of immunocytes and immunoglobulin producers we are obviously moving into specifically immunological territory, and before applying a similar dynamic approach to functionally active immunocytes it is logically necessary to consider modern theories of immunity.

CHAPTER 3

Modern immunological theory

In 1972 it is possible to characterize modern immunology as being based on the reactions of cells that on differentiation become capable of synthesizing one particular type of antibody or immunoglobulin. This has as its primary function to serve as a receptor which will allow each cell to react specifically to contact with an appropriate antigenic determinant. It is convenient to speak of such cells as immunocytes and to concentrate initially on the antibodies they produce.

The nature of antibodies

Antibodies are proteins usually studied in the form of a soluble constituent of the circulating blood plasma, each molecular species of which can unite specifically with a certain chemical configuration which we call an antigenic determinant. The specificity of such union depends on the steric pattern of the determinant. This is a region, usually part of a larger molecule or particle, whose size can be roughly stated as equivalent to that of three to six amino acid or hexose residues in protein or polysaccharide respectively. When the determinant can be obtained as an individual, small, molecular species, it is known as a hapten. In general, such molecules can block the activity of the corresponding antibody to a recognizable extent. They are, however, not immunogenic in the sense that they fail to provoke an antibody response when administered to an animal and give at most a very incomplete non-precipitating reaction with the corresponding antibody. Specificity as between antigenic determinant and antibody is far from absolute. Usually a number of broadly similar chemical configurations will react with a single antibody but show a wide range in the affinity of union. Chemically, antibodies can be classed as one or other of five main types of immunoglobulin known as IgG, IgM, IgA, IgD, and IgE. The commonest of these, IgG, is subdivided into four subclasses in man and has more or less equivalent complexity in other species.

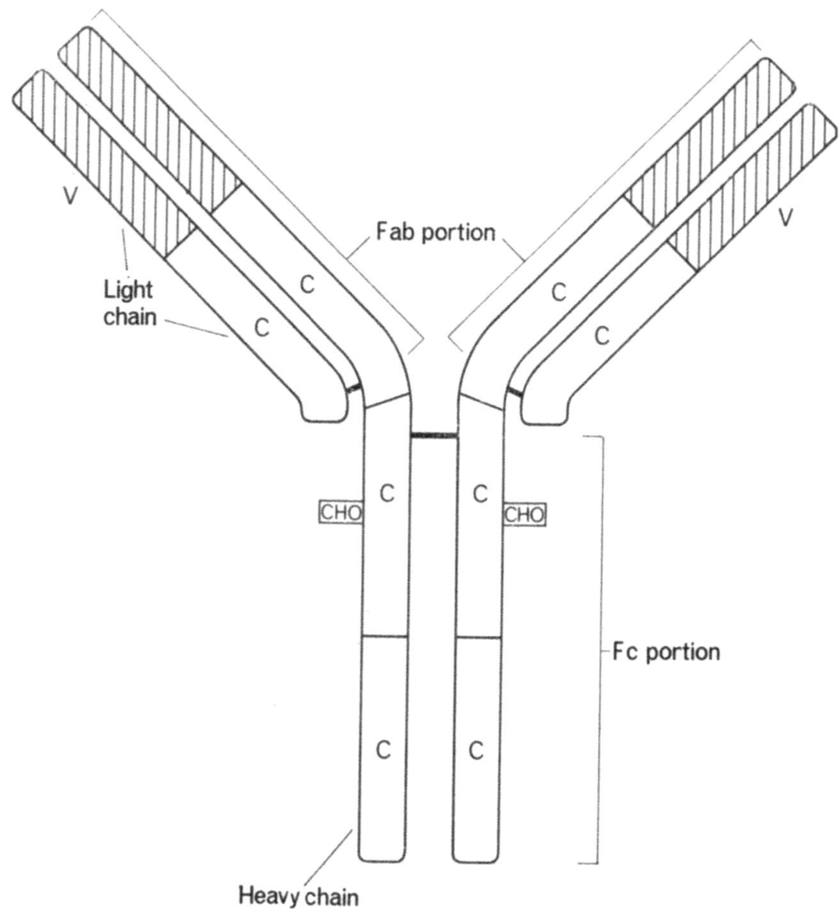

FIG. 8. Modified Porter's diagram for IgG. Each heavy chain is made up of four units, three constant and one variable, while each light chain has one constant and one variable unit. The variable units are shaded and their interaction gives rise to the two similar combining sites with which antigenic determinants react. Interchain disulphide bonds are shown by heavy lines; the disposition of Fab and Fc fractions obtained by enzyme action, and the approximate site of the carbohydrate moiety CHO, are also indicated.

Any discussion of the structure of antibody must be based on that of a typical IgG antibody and make use of a slightly modernized version of R. R. Porter's diagram (Fig. 8). Such an antibody is a complex protein of molecular weight, around 155,000, built up of four polypeptide chains held together by three disulphide bonds; it also includes two carbohydrate units (oligosaccharides containing mannose, galactose, glucosamine, fucose, and sialic acid). The molecule is a symmetrical one with two light chains (L) of 214± amino acid residues and two heavy chains (H), each of approximately twice the size. There is now unanimity that each light chain is made up of two segments, each of 107 residues, the one at the N-terminal end being known as the variable segment (V), while the other is the constant segment (C). The heavy chain has four homologous segments of which the N-terminal one is variable and the other three constant.

The terms 'variable' and 'constant' refer simply to the results of comparing the corresponding segments of a large number of pure antibodies of the same immunoglobulin type. With modern methods devised largely by Edman, the sequence of amino acids in any peptide chain can be established. In the constant segments each antibody shows the same sequence except for an occasional instance where one or other of two different amino acids can occupy the same position. In the variable segment, however, there is a general resemblance in the pattern of sequence, but many differences in detail from one antibody to another. Some short regions of a variable segment show many more sequence differences than others and are spoken of as hypervariable. The variable segments of L and H chains are associated, as shown in the diagram, and each L–H(V) pair gives rise to the combining site which determines the specificity of the antibody. The two combining sites on the molecule each have the same specificity and are determined by the amino acid sequences of the two variable segments and the three-dimensional configuration that they develop. Enormous numbers of different sequences are available amongst the variable segments and the range of possible combining site patterns, and therefore of antibody patterns, is almost unlimited.

The mass of recent work on amino acid sequences of the immunoglobulin chains has introduced many complexities which are hardly relevent to clinical and biological discussion of auto-immune disease. For our purposes the most important features of the immunoglobulins in man are as follows:

1. All immunoglobulins have light chains of the same character.

2. The types G, M, A, D, and E are based on the antigenic character of the heavy chains, but there are also physical differences. IgM in mammals is approximately five times larger than IgG and can be

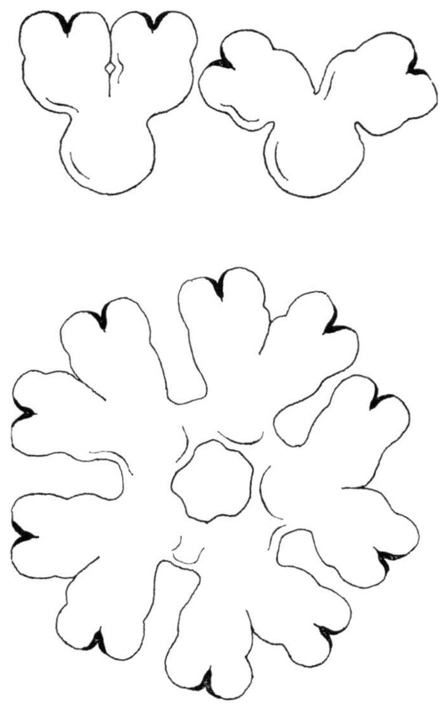

FIG. 9. Semidiagrammatic sketches to indicate the probable shape of molecules of IgG and IgM. Note the flexibility of the molecule in the two configurations of IgG. Position of the combining sites is indicated by thickened line. (Burnet and White, *Natural History of Infectious Disease*, 4th edition, Cambridge University Press, 1972.)

regarded as a pentamer, held together by disulphide bonds, of a structure closely similar to an IgG molecule.

3. In man there are two antigenic types of light chain, κ and λ; these are present in a ratio of about 2:1 respectively in all individuals. Within each type there are three subtypes based on amino acid sequences.

4. Immunoglobulins G, M, A, and D are present in all individuals in that order of frequency. IgE is probably always present but is only conspicuous in allergic subjects.

The diversity of immune patterns

At the level of molecular biology, interest in immunoglobulins centres on the genetic and biochemical processes by which a wide diversity of antibodies can be created, sufficient to deal with almost any foreign organic configuration that can be introduced into the body. The earlier idea that each antibody was made to order to fit any foreign antigen that might intrude into the antibody-producing cell has gone for ever. Each antibody pattern is directly determined by the standard genetically guided process of protein synthesis. The diversity is generated at the genetic level. Each immunocyte carries receptors with combining sites of antibody quality and is stimulated to proliferate or to produce antibody of a particular Ig type by specific contact with antigenic determinants which have adequate binding affinity for the combining site of the receptor.

For fairly obvious reasons much more investigation has been focused on antibody than on immunocytes and for not so obvious reasons even more on myeloma proteins than on normal antibodies. In a brief outline there is no call to follow the history of how immunological ideas developed. It is simpler and more satisfactory to accept the current teaching and use this to interpret the virtues of the various approaches. In a nutshell, the accepted doctrine is that, by a process that I have often likened to the generation of random four-letter words by a computer, a genetic process still far from adequately understood develops the capacity to specify a very large number of 'combining site patterns' as well as five distinct types and an uncertain number of subtypes of immunoglobulin on which to impress such patterns. At a certain stage of stem cell development, some time before differentiation to an immunocyte occurs, an internal decision is made as to the type and specificity of the immunoglobulin it will produce. There are two rules. The first is that the cell and any descendants it may have will produce only one type of immunoglobulin carrying one, and only one, pattern of specific reactivity which it is convenient to call immune pattern. This is the rule of phenotypic restriction which can be accepted as virtually absolute. No cell, however, is immune from the possibility of mutation and there is evidence that rarely a plasma cell line may mutate to give an altered antibody product. In addition it now appears that IgM-producing clones may under some circumstances switch to become IgG-producers. The possibility is still open that at a certain stage of differentiation all types of immunoglobulin producers synthesize IgM, sometimes in monomeric rather than in the classical pentameric form. The change to G, A, D, or E then becomes a secondary change in which the original light chain and the variable heavy segment remain unchanged, so preserving the antibody specificity of the cell line.

The second rule is that the source of diversity of immune pattern is powerful enough to ensure an almost random distribution of patterns and an effective diversity. There is no possibility of proving the statement, but intuitively I should expect that if we could check a large population of cells for the amino acid sequence in the combining sites of each immunocyte's receptor and antibody immediately the decision had been made and phenotypic restriction applied, we should find an effectively infinite variety. If the first differentiated cell has pattern A, then it may be many thousands of cells later before immune pattern A appears on differentiation.

There are, however, conceptual difficulties in ascribing the whole diversity of antibody pattern to a completely random mechanism. Genetic processes in the normal sense are undoubtedly deeply concerned in determining the structure of immunoglobulins. Probably most immunologists interested in this field would agree that an extensive range of genetic information relevant to antibody structure is present in the fertilized ovum. One common approach is to postulate a large number of related genes (initially arising by duplication), each corresponding to one of the 100–20 amino acid segments from which all immunoglobulins seem to be built. In principle, a large variety of antibody and immunoglobulin patterns could be produced by simple assortment of the genetic units in different combinations. There are some antibodies (as cell receptors) which seem to be produced in unusually large amount, and Jerne has suggested that these may be antibodies either built wholly to germ-line instructions or developed by some modification occurring with a high probability at an early stage. Some theorists, notably Hood, have suggested that there is nothing to exclude the possibility that *all* antibodies are determined in this simple genetic fashion, the only unique quality of the process being the extremely large number of alternate genes from which combinations can be built up.

The great majority of investigators, however, prefer to postulate a relatively small 'library' of germ-line genes that might produce a few hundred different antibodies and superimpose a process taking place in the stem cells as they mature, which can greatly expand diversity. According to some (Gally and Edelman), intragenomic interaction between genes, equivalent to recombination and crossing over, is responsible. Others postulate hyperactive mutation concentrated on what are now called the hyper-variable regions of the variable segments (Cohn, Milstein).

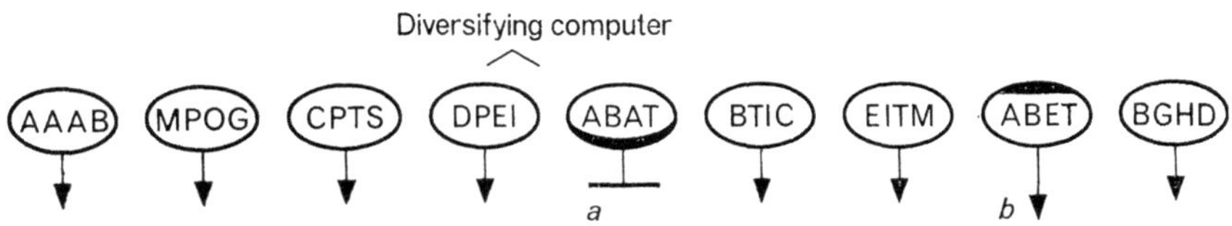

FIG. 10. A diagram to suggest the process by which antibody diversity is generated and appropriate patterns selected. A computer generates four-letter combinations at random.

a. Any combination recognizable as a French word (for example, abat), corresponds to a 'self' component and is eliminated.

b. Any English word (for example, abet) corresponds to an antigenic determinant of some micro-organism that may invade the body. When this happens, cells carrying the pattern will proliferate.

There is still no decisive evidence that favours one or the other theory and one senses a growing doubt as to whether any detailed interpretation in molecular-genetic terms will ever be possible. For our purposes it is probably adequate to assume that by the time of birth all mammals have generated a wide enough diversity of receptor and antibody patterns to function effectively and that the range of patterns available goes on extending probably at least to the stage of early adult life.

Work with pure line animals has shown that there are considerable differences between strains of mice or guinea pigs in their ability to produce antibody against some synthetic peptide antigens. At least some of these failures to produce antibody are due not to any inability to synthesize the necessary immune pattern but to genetic differences in capacity to carry out one or more of the processes that are needed to allow expression of the immunogenicity of the antigenic determinant-carrier complex being used. Having due regard to all the factors which may be needed, in addition to antibody-like immune receptors, before antibody production or the development of delayed hypersensitivity can be experimentally demonstrated, there is little justification for speculating about what patterns are actually inherited. To use teleological language, nature's objective is to use a randomization mechanism to produce as comprehensive a repertoire of immune patterns as is possible with the material that is available. If we program a computer to produce 100,000 four-letter 'words' at random from the normal alphabet, we might find on scanning the result that 100 were accepted English words. On running several such programs, the 100± English words that emerged would differ widely from one set to another. All sorts of relevant modifications could be considered to increase the output of English words (equivalent to potentially useful antibody patterns) in ways that could be compared with what in the immunological system might have happened in the course of evolution. The numbers of each letter in the pool could be proportional to its use in English: E > T > A > I, etc. Rules could be put into the program that any sequence of consonants or vowels must be no longer than two or that a large number of binary combinations of consonants are forbidden. Still using wholly random selection, such program modifications might ensure that in every run of 100,000 random four-letter words at least 95 per cent of those existing in current English would be produced. Without attempting to suggest any details whatever of the evolutionary programming, I believe that anyone with some knowledge of protein structure and its evolution and synthesis will recognize the relevance of the analogy.

Diversification of immune pattern is a random process carried out within a framework of rules. Some of the rules are known or can be guessed at intelligently, most are unknown. One pictures the diversification proceeding wholly at the genetic level, i.e. without any form of phenotypic expression, through most of embryonic development.

For the present purpose the significant point is that if random processes are responsible for the nature of the immune pattern that a newly differentiated immunocyte will express, *large numbers of those cells will carry a pattern complementary to and reactive with potential antigenic determinants present in the body.*

On this basis one can offer certain summarized points about immune pattern diversity which are relevant to auto-immune disease. In the first place, having regard to the disposition of 20 different types of amino acid in antibody-combining sites with a significant length of 10–20 amino acid residues on each of the 2 variable segments, it is possible to have an effectively infinite variety of immune patterns. This holds even if, as is undoubtedly the case, some amino acid replacements would render the combining site non-functional.

The second point is essentially a warning against the persisting influence of 'instructive' theories of antibody formation which were universally current until recently. It is very easy to adopt semi-unconsciously the idea that there is a unique relationship between the antigenic determinant and the antibody combining site of the particular antigen–antibody combination one happens to be working with. This is a dangerous attitude; the situation is much more soft-edged. Suppose we consider a chemically defined antigenic determinant: a dinitrophenyl (DNP) group, for instance, on a standard carrier protein. In an immunized rabbit there will be much anti-DNP antibody whose reactivity with the synthetic hapten can be shown in various ways. That antibody is not, however, chemically homogeneous. It is composed of a heterogeneous collection of immunoglobulin molecules whose only common feature is that the immune pattern of their combining sites is such that they will combine with the antigenic determinant with a degree of affinity which will allow the union to contribute to a detectable effect. Perhaps the significance of this is best shown by contrasting the proportion of immunoglobulin molecules of graded degrees of affinity for union with DNP (*a*) in a normal serum, (*b*) in serum from an immunized animal in two histograms. We assume arbitrarily eight grades of affinity, bearing in mind that there are few proteins which will not adsorb almost any organic substance to some extent at least.

We could equally produce a similar diagram by considering a pure population of molecules of antibody, for example, from one of the not uncommon myeloma proteins which react with DNP. It is known that such a population, when tested with DNP, shows a standard value for affinity of union. If, however, we take a large series of nitro-phenyl and similar aromatic compounds which can be used as haptens and test their affinity, many will be found to show significant binding power; some almost certainly would show a 'better fit' and higher affinity than the DNP used in detecting the reactive myeloma protein in the first place.

This may seem a ponderous way of emphasizing the 'soft edge' of immunological reactions, but I feel that it is essential to grasp the point if auto-immune disease is to be understood. It means simply that the specificity of any individual antigen–antibody interaction is far from being as unique as it used to be assumed when 'instructive' theories of antibody production held sway.

The third point is merely to transfer the same argument to those immune patterns, carried by newly differentiated immunocytes, which can react with some potential antigenic determinant in the body. There are, of course, many thousand potential antigenic determinants in the soluble proteins of the blood plasma and many more which are accessible on the surface of circulating and endothelial cells in contact with the plasma. For any single antigenic determinant we

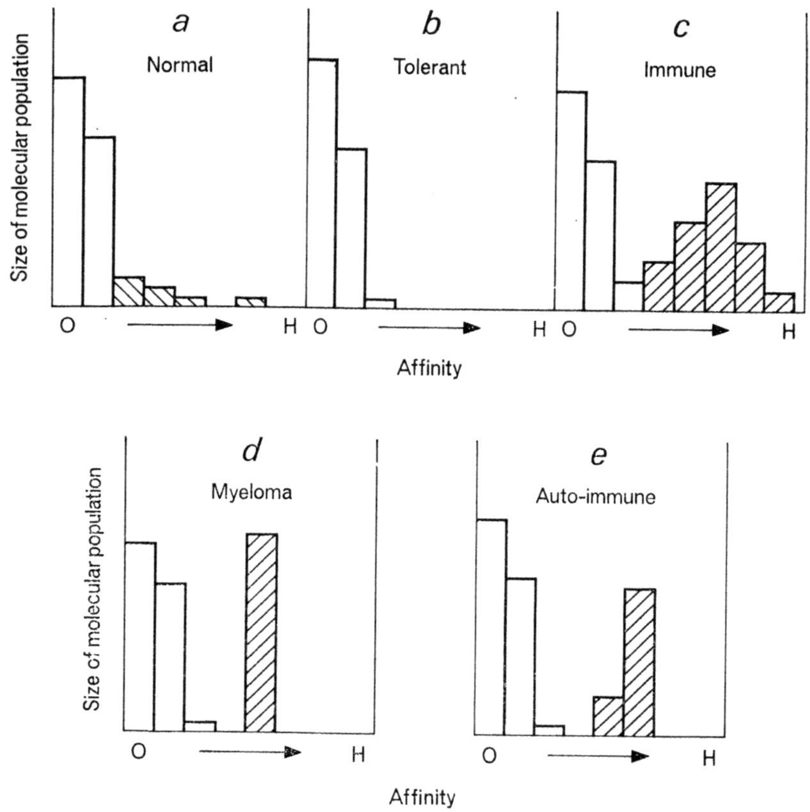

FIG. 11. The distribution of reactivity with a single antigenic determinant amongst immunocyte populations present in individuals of different immunological status. In each section a series of histograms indicating the relative size of molecular populations of antibody or of immunocytes in terms of their immune (antibody-like) receptors, sorted into eight grades of affinity, from zero (o) to high (H), for a given antigenic determinant. Shaded histograms indicate the presence of significant immune activity by conventional criteria.

a–c. Showing normal, tolerant, and immune individuals. The AD is assumed to be one foreign to the body and in principle the histograms can be applied to circulating antibody at the molecular level or to either T- or B-immunocytes in terms of their immune receptors. Note that if an AD natural to, and accessible in, the body is considered, the situation shown as 'tolerant' obtains in all normal individuals.

d–e. Similar figures for pathological conditions. For myeloma there is a uniform population of one level of affinity for any AD which may be reactive. In an auto-immune situation the AD is of self-origin and the situation must be compared with 'tolerant' in *a–c*. In general, many fewer clones will be involved in an auto-immune situation than in simple immunization by a foreign antigen.

could probably construct a figure broadly similar to Fig. 11 (normal). Its significance would be that, other things being equal, immunocytes with affinities 1, 2, and 3 could be tolerated as harmless; the occasional cell with affinity in the upper range from 5 to 8 is a potential initiator of an auto-immune clone and must be inhibited from multiplication or destroyed. This is the essence of immunological tolerance and its further discussion can be deferred to a separate chapter on that topic.

Population dynamics of immunocytes

Turning now to cellular aspects of immunology and picking up the story of population dynamics of the circulating cells derived from bone marrow, we need first to say something more about primary differentiation to immunocytes. The orthodox viewpoint is that at some point a line of stem cells without capacity to respond to antigen is differentiated in the sense that from that point onward all descendants of what can now be called an immunocyte will produce a specifically defined immunoglobulin expressed as receptor or as liberated antibody. On this assumption the whole process of intragenomic recombination, mutation, and 'choice' of one particular pattern for expression must have taken place amongst the cell lines leading from fertilized ovum to the stem cells of bone marrow. The stimulus to expression of the immunoglobulin under phenotypic restriction was ascribed in part to the thymus, in part to some undefined region of lymphoid tissue in mammals presumed to be homologous to the bursa of Fabricius in birds.

There is a wide range of support from competent investigators for such an outline, but it is undoubtedly an over-simplification and it may be basically incorrect. There are still quite conflicting opinions as to where the first differentiation, definable as when immunoglobulin receptors can first be demonstrated on the cell surface, takes place. The stimulus to differentiation must be more subtle than simple lodgement in a particular micro-environment, and in fact the apparent role of thymus seems to vary considerably from one mammalian species to another. No one has produced even an interesting theory as to how the various cell lines which will produce the different immunoglobulins G, M, A, D, and E are differentiated. Equally, no one interested in the immunological character of the mouse thymus has offered any explanation of how under some circumstances large areas of cortex can undergo what seems to be an autocatalytic conversion to mast cells.

And there has been a tendency to say little about the experiments by which labelled thoracic duct lymphocytes can apparently be transformed to Kupfer cells or in which they give rise to peritoneal macrophages. Possibly even more important is it to note the increasing number of minor and major genetic anomalies of immune function that are being observed in man. Many of these involve immunoglobulins and capacity to produce antibody, and very few of them have been fitted into any consistent theory of immunocyte differentiation.

Everywhere one finds a soft edge in experiments designed to follow the fate of a given population and one is more and more inclined to look for stochastic regularities rather than determinative ones. In the last analysis the only thing we may be able to say is that in the mature functional form we can identify three major groups: (1) immunocytes, (2) plasma cells producing IgG, M, A, D, or E, and (3) mast cells. At some point each clone must have arisen from a stem cell, but we may be able to say no more than to suggest that a stem cell has a certain probability of adopting the role of every one of those types, the relative proportions being appropriate to functional need. Once a role has been adopted, i.e. once the cell has differentiated, a phenotypic restriction operates so that all descendant cells (or at least the great majority) breed true. It is well established that some IgM-producing cells switch to IgG production, while others do not, and other rarer interchanges may well take place even if so far they have never been experimentally recognized.

In the mouse it appears highly probable that for cells to manifest the functions we speak of as thymus-dependent they must either spend some time as a developing clone within the thymus or be subject to some hormone liberated by the thymus. Yet unexpected happenings are legion. Standard Swiss mice (which are not a pure line strain) show for a period after neonatal thymectomy the expected incapacity to reject foreign skin grafts. They do not, however, show the 'runting' and death observed in many pure line strains after about three months, and by the time they are fully grown their immune capacity is not demonstrably inferior to that of mice which have retained their thymuses. It is almost more disconcerting to find that sheep thymectomized halfway through gestation are born with hardly any immune deficiency.

It must never be forgotten that one nucleus differs from another not in the potential information it contains but in the portion of it which is in a derepressed condition. A little is known about the *lac*-operon functions in bacteria, but virtually nothing about how differentiation is controlled in embryonic mammalian cells or in stem cells during post-natal life. Most of the controversies amongst cytologists interested in the phenomena of infection, inflammation, and immunity are concerned with whether cell *B* is or is not derived from a cell of type *A*. Many such difficulties may never be resolved and we may have to be content with some reasonable extrapolations from whatever model experimental system seems to us the most logically or aesthetically attractive. Probably the most important thing to remember is that even if some unusual switch by a cell from one type of phenotypic expression to another is excessively rare, any circumstances which provoke proliferation of the new derivative may make it quite conspicuous. It is probably not far from the truth to say that any type of somatic cell can be transformed into any other type, but the probabilities of each change differ enormously.

If we accept this stochastic approach it provides an explanation of the soft edges of all experiments and may well suggest that a very large proportion of experimental work is of no significance to anything but the specific situation being investigated. It also engenders a certain scepticism about the significance of results obtained in such biological monstrosities as pure line mice neonatally thymectomized, lethally irradiated, and salvaged by injection of bone marrow from another mouse. Many unsuspected things could be happening in those mutilated mice.

The role of the thymus

The position of the thymus is crucial to any understanding of the population dynamics of lymphocytes. Most of the work has been done in mice and the following description is based primarily on this species. There is a constant entry of cells from the blood into the thymus, circumstantial evidence pointing strongly to the bone marrow as the origin of the stem cells. The entering cells proliferate for approximately 10–12 days and the progeny then disappear from the thymus. Many are killed *in situ*, but in the neonatal mouse or hamster large numbers are released into the circulation and serve to colonize the peripheral lymph nodes, spleen, and other lymphoid accumulations. The number escaping from the thymus diminishes sharply as the animal grows. In general the long-lived, circulating lymphocytes are thymus-dependent in the sense that they are diminished or absent in neonatally thymectomized mice. This leaves open the possibility that only a small proportion of thymus-dependent, or T-, cells have actually spent any time in the thymus; the others are descendants of cells which have.

The most definitive recent approach has been to use refined methods of detecting antigens and immunoglobulin on the lymphocyte surface. There is agreement that immunoglobulins are not seen on cortical lymphocytes from the thymus. These cells, however, develop a series of specific antigens, some of which persist when descendants of these cells become circulating lymphocytes. According to Boyse (1970), thymocytes (i.e. lymphocytes in the thymic cortex) carry at least six sorts of surface antigen in mice, each with its own genetic locus. Most of them show antigenic specificities that vary from strain to strain, corresponding to allelomorphic genes. The antigens are TL, found only on thymocytes, θ on thymocytes and in reduced amount on a proportion of circulating lymphocytes, and H2, the standard histocompatibility antigen, found on all cells of the animal. Two other antigenic structures are not well understood and can be omitted from discussion.

The proportion of lymphocytes carrying immunoglobulin varies according to the species of animal and the sensitivity of the test used to detect the relevant antigens. In mice it is generally accepted that cells with TL or θ do not show immunoglobulin when tested by methods making use of immunofluorescence. Those which do show readily demonstrated immunoglobulin are B-cells (see p. 49), from which antibody-secreting plasma cells are derived and which carry another specific surface antigen, Pca. In the rabbit, however, using a sensitive technique Pernis has evidence that the proportion of lymphocytes carrying immunoglobulin must include some that by other criteria would be classed as T-immunocytes. There are other indications that (*a*) stem cells lacking θ or TL antigen develop these in the thymus and (*b*) cells derived from the thymus lose the TL antigen after some time in the circulation.

The most likely interpretation is that the thymic influence, inducing differentiation to or toward immunocyte function, is of hormonal nature and secreted by the thymic epithelial cells. It is most effective when the thymocytes are actually in the thymus, but there is evidence that cells can develop 'thymus-dependent' activity by exposure to products of thymic epithelium growing as grafts or in 'millipore' chambers. Recent work suggests that a relatively low molecular weight substance, 'thymosin', may be responsible for the effect.

Multiple myeloma and myeloma proteins

Like almost every other type of cell in the body, immunocytes are subject to malignant change, and since one of the main objectives of this book is to draw attention to the resemblances of the auto-immune process to malignant disease, some consideration of myelomatosis is called for. This disease can be regarded as a low-grade malignancy involving immunocytes of the immunoglobulin-producing series, i.e. plasmablasts or immature plasma cells. For the immunologist this disease is of the greatest interest, particularly because it can be induced with some regularity in at least one strain of mice, as well as being a not very uncommon human ailment, especially in elderly men. Quite regularly the blood plasma of such patients contains an excess of immunoglobulin produced by cells of the myeloma clone and in the great majority the immunoglobulin represents a population of identical molecules. In Waldenström's phrase, it is a monoclonal dysgammaglobulinaemia.

There are two aspects of myelomatosis that are of special interest in the present context. The first is its monoclonal character. In view of the enormous variety of immunoglobulin molecules present in any normal human serum, the strict uniformity of the myeloma protein means that all the cells concerned form part of a clone derived from a *single cell* in which some initiating process which we can speak of as a somatic mutation took place. There may be a variety of other malignant conditions involving stem cell derivatives which are equally monoclonal (leukaemias, Hodgkin's disease, lymphosarcoma, and so on) but there is not the same convenient criterion available that there is with myeloma.

The second aspect emerges when a large number of myeloma globulins, each from a different patient, are compared. Every one is unique and over-all they comprise examples of all the immunoglobulins G, M, A, D, and E and of all the common sub-types of G. Both κ and λ types of light chain are found. What is of special interest is that the proportion of the different types and sub-types found in a large collection of such myeloma proteins corresponds closely to the proportion of each immunoglobulin that would be found in pooled serum from a group of normal individuals of the same racial and regional origin. The implication is that any immature plasma cell is equally liable to suffer the initiating episode at some extremely low frequency: a frequency that I once calculated, using some very arbitrary assumptions, might be of the order of 10^{-20} per cell generation.

A third point arises here. With that extreme rarity it is inconceivable that any individual would develop two independent myeloma clones. This is seen only in less than 0·5 per cent of cases and when it occurs must *a priori* be ascribed to secondary change occurring within the proliferating clone. In Fudenberg's laboratory Wang *et al.* (1970) have described one such case in which both M and G immunoglobulins were present and where both proteins carried apparently identical light chains: a strong indication that the two clones derived from a single primary mutation.

Finally it should be mentioned that myeloma proteins are found in the serum of two different classes of hospital patient. There are those with classical multiple myelomatosis, with focal lesions in the bone marrow which erode the bone and often result in spontaneous fractures. The second group are those patients, usually elderly men, who are detected by a detailed haematological examination made during the course of a 'diagnostic work-up'. The majority of such patients show no further development, some develop amyloid disease, and some go on to the classical picture of multiple myelomatosis with tumours in the bone marrow. Even a basically malignant condition can clearly be kept under an effective degree of control.

All four points will be found to be highly relevant to the discussion of auto-immune disease. Though it will have to be discussed in detail later it should be mentioned here that in some IgM monoclonal conditions the myeloma protein (the macroglobulin) has the specific character of an auto-antibody against immunoglobulin. This has the interesting implication that plasma cells of this specificity are sufficiently common in elderly people to serve occasionally as the initiating cell of the abnormal clone.

T and B immune systems

Today's central position in immunology of the dichotomy between T and B immune systems is a recent development and it is not impossible that it is only a temporary one. For the time being, however, it is of major importance in the understanding of auto-immune disease. For many years it has been known that delayed hypersensitivity reactions, Mantoux reaction to tuberculin for instance, were not associated with antibodies and were referred to as cell-mediated reactions in contrast to those dependent on antibody. Then in the 1950s it was recognized that in the immune deficiency disease, congenital agammaglobulinaemia, the patients, while incapable of producing antibody, nevertheless handled such a complex immunological process as an attack of measles with subsequent firm immunity just as competently as a normal individual. They rejected foreign skin grafts, albeit more slowly than normal, and developed delayed hypersensitivity reactions according to normal rules. Soon afterwards it was discovered that elimination of the bursa of Fabricius, either by surgery at hatching or by treatment with testosterone or equivalent hormones during incubation, left young chickens in approximately the same state as the child with agammaglobulinaemia.

The current doctrine to account for these findings is based essentially on two types of study. Very largely under the influence of R. A. Good, agammaglobulinaemia and a variety of other anomalies of immune response seen in new-born infants have been intensively investigated. Two of the conditions fit well into the categories of (*a*) complete absence of the B system (agammaglobulinaemia) and (*b*) failure of the thymus to develop with complete absence of the T system (DiGeorge's disease). The second source has been the investigations of J. F. A. P. Miller on the effects of neonatal thymectomy in mice. Thanks to Miller, the situation in CBA mice and their hybrids has been almost completely clarified during a decade of productive work. Broadly, the two groups of workers have reached similar conclusions and these will be the basis of the present discussion. As I have already hinted, however, investigations with other types of laboratory animal have differed in important aspects. There are several immunological anomalies of apparent genetic origin in man which do not fit at all comfortably in a simple B and T scheme. I feel reasonably confident that the current B and T formulation will be replaced within ten years by something more complex and flexible, but for the present it must be adopted mainly because in no other species of mammal has the situation been so intensively and effectively studied as in Miller's CBA mice.

Miller's current interpretation (Miller *et al.*, 1971) is approximately as follows. The circulating lymphocytes in mice can be divided into two sorts, which I shall call B- and T-immunocytes. The B-cells are antibody producers when converted into plasma cells by antigenic stimulation. They appear to be differentiated to immunocytes soon after leaving the bone marrow, but the site and circumstances are unknown.

B-lymphocytes and plasma cells have plentiful immunoglobulin patches on the cell membrane and no θ antigen.

T-immunocytes make up 80–90 per cent of the lymphocytes in thoracic duct lymph; they are derived ultimately from the bone marrow, but stem cells must spend two or three weeks at least proliferating in the thymic cortex before descendant T-immunocytes appear in the circulation. They have a characteristic antigen θ and, in mice, only the amount of immunoglobulin needed to provide receptors for immunological function. The evidence points strongly toward the T-cell receptor being composed of a monomeric IgM of approximately the same size as an IgG antibody molecule, but with the antigenic quality of IgM heavy chain. Another point of practical importance is that T-cells and not B-lymphocytes are stimulated to blast transformation and mitosis by phytohaemagglutinin (PHA). When anti-mouse lymphocyte serum is produced by standard methods in rabbits it is cytotoxic in the presence of complement for T- but not for B-lymphocytes or plasma cells. In guinea pigs and man at least, antigenic stimulation of T-cells results in their liberation of a variety of pharmacologically active substances which Dumonde calls 'lymphokines'.

Antibody, at least IgM and IgG antibody, is produced and liberated in significant amounts only by cells of the B system, predominantly by plasma cells but also by cells which could be called medium and large lymphocytes and blasts. B memory cells, i.e. cells and their descendants, morphologically lymphocytes, which can respond to a subsequent antigenic stimulus with a secondary type antibody response, are also produced when primary B-immunocytes are stimulated by antigen. Though Miller is not yet wholly convinced, the great majority of immunologists would accept the dogma that the pattern of antibody liberated by a B-cell is determined only by genetic processes in the ancestral line of the cell and that transfer of genetic information from another cell plays no part.

Co-operation of T- and B-cells in antibody production

In the last four years Miller's work has been largely concerned with the necessity for interaction between T- and B-cells if certain types of antibody are to be produced. Two very commonly used types of antigen, foreign red cells and semi-purified foreign serum proteins, can produce significant amounts of antibody in heavily irradiated mice only if both B- and T-cells are supplied. The evidence indicates that both types of cell must have specific receptors for the antigen if they are to co-operate effectively. There are other antigens, mostly micro-organismal, such as pneumococcal polysaccharide, *Salmonella* flagellin, or influenza virus, which do not require co-operation of T-immunocytes. The currently popular suggestion which best fits the facts is that these thymus-independent antigens all carry many identical antigenic determinants, making it easy for several antigenic determinants on the same particle or macromolecule to make contact with B receptors on a single B-cell. This is not characteristic of the soluble protein and cell surface antigens for which co-operation of T-cells is needed in order to induce proliferation of B-cells and antibody production.

Apart from the fact that both T- and B-cells must have specific receptors for the antigen, the nature of the co-operation is still obscure. A number of ingenious suggestions have been made, but I am not convinced that anything more is needed than to assume that when both T- and B-cells are present with the corresponding antigen in the same micro-environment the 'lymphokines' liberated by stimulated T-cells can activate what would otherwise be a sub-threshold antigenic stimulus for B into an effective one. When a simple hapten such as DNP is rendered immunogenic by being coupled chemically to a protein such as a foreign serum albumin which is then spoken of as carrier, it can be shown that antibody (produced by B-cells) is mostly anti-hapten while tests for cell-mediated responses (by T-cells) show specificity for the carrier. How far this is relevant in natural circumstances and in auto-immune disease will require later discussion.

Primary function of T-cells

The T-immunocyte has more important functions than as an adjuvant to antibody production and most of them are concerned with the liberation at the appropriate time and place of pharmacologically active agents which can stimulate and damage adjacent cells. For reasons which are too slender to justify elaboration I believe that the T system of immunocytes will eventually be divided into a number of subgroups on the basis of the types of lymphokine produced. Miller has already some evidence that I would interpret as showing that some T-cells produce lymphokines which stimulate other T-cells to more effective activity in graft versus host reactions.

At the experimental level the functional activity of T-cells is assessed by skin reactivity of delayed hypersensitivity (DH) type. This is legitimately taken as a prototype of all cell-mediated immunity. DH reactions are specific, but specificity is at a much lower level than antibody specificity, for example, flagellins from two distinct *Salmonellas*, *S. adelaide* and *S. typhimurium*, provoke quite distinct antibodies, but DH reactions induced by one are about equal for both flagellins. Similar cross-reactivity in DH tests can be seen with synthetic antigens.

As in so many other areas of experimental immunology, detailed discussion needs almost always to be limited to one species of animal and one particular range of antigens. Any attempt at broader coverage is only possible in very general biological terms. Without attempting to forecast any future subtleties of approach we can look on T-cells as primarily being concerned with the removal of *cells* whose surfaces are recognized as alien. This holds for surgically implanted foreign tissue grafts, for tumours initiated in the body and for cells viably infected by viruses. In all probability, modifications of cell surfaces by chemical substances, from beryllium, nickel, and zirconium salts to poison ivy, may equally call for handling by T-cells or one of their subgroups. One pictures the general process as one in which the foreign configuration from the cell surface is carried to the local lymph node, most probably loosely incorporated in the surface of a wandering lymphocyte or monocyte. Once contact is made with an appropriate T-immunocyte this is stimulated to multiply and to stimulate other unrelated cells to proliferate. Eventually the specific T-cells and non-specifically proliferated 'newborn' lymphocytes of other lines reach the foreign target cells. Cytotoxic substances are released and there is extensive cellular destruction of specific immunocytes, other lymphocytes, target cells, and adjacent normal cells. Biologically, only the death and disposal of the target cells are of any significance. Once that has been accomplished, dead and damaged cells of all types can be easily handled like any other piece of traumatized tissue.

One feature of special significance is that there is a strong indication that antigenic stimulation of a T-immunocyte can set in train something of a chain reaction. The lymphokines can act on other lymphocytes non-specifically in approximately the same fashion as an antigenic stimulus acts on a T-immunocyte, including liberation of new lymphokines. This provides a typically biological expedient to multiply the capacity of a small number of specific cells to attack the target tissue.

Whenever in auto-immune disease we find destructive infiltration of a tissue with lymphocytes we can be confident that specifically active T-immunocytes are concerned. But it is characteristic of the complexity of everything living that there will usually be some obvious plasma cells and one can be equally certain that many of the lymphocytes are casual participants without specific auto-immune quality.

The functions of antibody

Twenty years ago antibody was given the credit for recovery from every infectious disease or localized infection and those who believed in auto-immune disease assumed that antibody was responsible for any damaging effect in such conditions. Amongst the other charges in immunological opinion since the early 1950s has been a striking demotion of antibody from its position at the centre of the stage. The behaviour of children with agammaglobulinaemia, who have no capacity to produce antibody, has been largely responsible for this. The facts that such children show the normal signs and symptoms of measles and recover with long-lasting immunity and that they respond normally to Jennerian vaccination have been specially impressive. The major weakness is an incapacity to resist bacterial infection, and before the days of antibiotics all such children probably died from pneumonia at an early age. With regular small injections of normal human immunoglobulins and careful watch for and control of infection, many of the children enjoy reasonable health and one must assume that a variety of other immunological mechanisms are functioning effectively without benefit of actively produced antibody.

The defensive function of antibody seems to be almost limited to dealing with micro-organisms found extracellularly, particularly bacteria. There can be no doubt about the importance of the opsonizing function in the elimination of bacterial infection or of the value of antitoxin production when this is relevant. It is also hard to believe that antibody is not the effective protecting agent in immunity to arthropod-borne virus infections.

There is a growing feeling that one of the main functions of antibody is to prevent any excessive impact of antigen on the immune mechanism. Quite minute amounts of antigen can be effective as a stimulus to proliferation of the corresponding immunocytes and large amounts are liable to destroy or inhibit them (high zone tolerance). Most of the bacteria opsonized by antibody and phagocytosed by polymorphonuclear leucocytes or macrophages are effectively removed as antigen from the system. In similar fashion, if a soluble antigenic particle is coated with antibody it is incapable of specifically stimulating immunocyte receptors.

It can probably be accepted that whenever a typical micro-organismal infection occurs there is specific stimulation of both T- and B-immunocytes, not necessarily by the same sets of antigenic determinants. It can be expected in fact that a very complex story will be uncovered when, if ever, the populations of specifically stimulated immunocytes are evaluated after a rabbit, say, is infected with a sub-lethal dose of *Salmonella* bacteria. It has already been indicated, for instance, that only antigens with repetitive identical determinants stimulate B-immunocytes with ease, and I have suggested that stimulation of T-immunocytes concerned in delayed hypersensitivity or homograft rejection is most readily achieved by antigenic determinants carried in the cell membrane of another body cell.

Nevertheless, one would guess that there are very many situations where both T- and B-immunocytes can be stimulated by the same antigenic determinant. When this is the case, the coexistence of antigen with antibody and reactive T- and B-immunocytes provides a situation in which competitive actions of various types can occur. In particular, free antibody is likely to unite with antigen whether this is free in body fluid or held non-specifically on some cell surface. When this happens the antigen is no longer able to stimulate either T- or B-cells to proliferate. Antibody thus acts as a negative feedback to inhibit its own continued production. Capacity to inhibit T-cells of the corresponding specificity is of even greater potential importance in relation to auto-immune disease. If a target cell surface antigen *X* has provoked both T and B responses, the antibody anti-*X* may be in a position to blanket *X* on the cells concerned so that they can act neither as stimulus to T-cell proliferation nor as recognizable targets for specific cytotoxic attack by existent T-immunocytes. In some circumstances, therefore, the presence of auto-antibody may prevent completely or partially inhibit auto-immune disease. Conversely, one of the reasons why arthritis with some resemblance to rheumatoid arthritis is so common in patients with agammaglobulinaemia may be because of the absence of the buffering effect of auto-antibodies. In similiar fashion, anti-tumour antibody may 'enhance' the transplantability of a tumour, presumably by preventing it from stimulating a T response.

An important practical application of this general principle is in the prevention of Rh disease (haemolytic disease of the new-born) which results from maternal production of antibody when during the process of birth small amounts of foetal blood pass into the mother's circulation. If such cells carry the 'positive Rh antigen' D, derived from the father, and the mother is Rh negative, i.e. has no antigen D, then she is likely to develop anti-D if the foreign cells remain in the circulation for any significant length of time. Two things may protect her. If the foetal cells are of an incompatible ABO group, for example, if the baby-to-be is type A and the mother type O, they will be coated with the mother's natural antibody and swept out of the way. If they are ABO compatible, an injection of a small amount of anti-D antibody at the time of birth of each child will serve equally well to prevent cells carrying the D antigen from provoking active formation of the unwanted anti-D.

Complexities of the situation

It should be clear from this discussion of T and B immune systems that the situation in man or any experimental mammal is extremely complex. Future investigation seems much more likely to introduce fresh complications than to produce a new clarification. Most of the functional studies of antibody production and T-cell function have used Jerne's method of recognizing and counting plaque-forming cells, i.e. cells capable of producing antibody against an undefined set of antigenic determinants on the foreign red cell surface, which when complement is added haemolyses the red cells. IgM and IgG antibodies can be differentiated and the only T-cells that are involved are those which need to co-operate with B-cells to induce them to synthesize and liberate antibody. No notice has been taken of cells producing immunoglobulins A, D, and E; the limitations of the switch with IgM producers to IgG producers are unknown. Miller has already indicated that there are two types of T-cell, which in itself implies that with appropriate new experimentation other subgroups would be defined. In the sheep, mid-gestational thymectomy has virtually no effect on any type of antibody production and does not modify homograft rejection. The only demonstrable effect in the lamb is to diminish the number of circulating lymphocytes and weaken, but not abolish, the capacity to develop delayed hypersensitivity. There is an evident paradox if in the sheep most T-cells are not thymus-dependent.

Yet other complexities emerge when foetal animals are intensively studied. So far this has only been possible in the sheep, which has a gestation of 150 days. At 65 days' foetal age bacteriophage and ferritin will produce antibody, at around 80 days skin homografts are rejected, at 120 days antibody to ovalbumin can be produced. Once initiated, each capacity persists, but not until some weeks after birth can antibodies be produced against diphtheria toxoid or a *Salmonella* vaccine. Foetal lambs thymectomized at 75 days show the same sequence of development of these different immunological capacities.

Depending on temperament and mood, one can either despair of ever devising and carrying out the experiments needed to give a comprehensive account on mammalian immune systems or one can rejoice that for all the foreseeable future there will be significant problems potentially soluble by experiment that will keep an endless sequence of immunologists happy.

There are two important aspects of immunology which may be relevant here. For an immune system to be constructed on the principles that have evolved for the purpose in vertebrates demands a considerable lability of genetic change at both germinal and somatic levels. It is only to be expected, therefore, that evolutionary change should be relatively rapid and that wide structural and functional differences could be found in different groups of mammals. Even in so fundamental a matter as the thymus we have a cervical thymus in the guinea-pig, thoracic in other placental mammals, and two thymuses, one cervical, one thoracic, in most Australian marsupials. The effect of neonatal thymectomy is notoriously variable as between species. There are differences in detail and sometimes quite massive differences between experimental and observational findings in the favourite animal for study: man, sheep, rabbit, guinea-pig, and mouse. In general, each experimentalist of status finds it advisable to confine his studies to a few pure lines of one species and to make no serious attempt to equate his findings with those of workers using a different species.

For very similar reasons of genetic and somatic genetic liability we could expect to find many pathological anomalies of immune function in man. Some of the rare, severe, and theoretically significant anomalies have already been mentioned, but the range of lesser anomalies is literally infinite. If we include the standard clinical allergies and minor forms of auto-immune reactions, there must be very few human beings without a genetic anomaly that at some time produces symptoms or signs of illness. Any comprehensive survey of adult hospital patients will show anomalies in the distribution of immunoglobulins, for example, absence or a gross deficiency of IgA. Almost every year a new type of inherited immunological abnormality is recognized and reported in some unfortunate infant. The auto-immune diseases in man with which all this discussion is primarily concerned are extremely diverse and difficult to fit into clear nosological divisions and, quite characteristically, virtually every sign or immune reaction that can be used to identify auto-immune disease will be found in a proportion of individuals without other evidence of disease.

This book is not concerned with allergy or with the gross immuno-deficiency diseases of genetic origin, and before we can attempt any analysis of auto-immune disease the nature of immunological tolerance must be discussed. It will add new depth and new complexities to the picture of the normal mechanisms of immunity.

CHAPTER 4

Tolerance and paralysis

As soon as immunologists began to use red blood cells or blood serum as experimental antigens it was recognized that an animal which could react strongly against red cells from another species gave no response against an injection of its own cells or in general against cells from another individual of the same species. On the simplest common-sense grounds, too, it was obvious that there must be some inbuilt inhibition preventing immune reactions against the body's own constituents. Ehrlich spoke of 'horror autotoxicus' as a general principle to cover this immunological distinction between self and not self. In discussing auto-immune disease we shall be concerned almost wholly with conditions where to some extent these normal inhibitions have broken down. The fact that auto-immune disease is rare in man and exceptionally rare in other animals merely underlines the importance of the inviolability of self-components.

The development of natural tolerance

On general grounds the simplest hypothesis might be that it is an inherited quality that immune responses are manifested against foreign cells and products but not against those genetically appropriate to the body. This can be excluded at once on the basis of those experiments which have shown that foreign cells (of the same species), if they are implanted at an appropriately early stage of embryonic life, can become established and persist indefinitely. They are tolerated immunologically in precisely the same way as cells genetically proper to the individual. The tolerance is something acquired during early life and not a genetic quality. The same must hold for the native tolerance of any vertebrate for its own cells or components. The fact that the healthy animal or man shows no evidence of immune attack, or of cells or antibodies capable of immune attack, against his own body constituents therefore demands a developmental and physiological interpretation, not a genetic one.

For obvious reasons no direct experiments are possible on the development of intrinsic tolerance in the normal animal. Theoretical interpretations have necessarily been developed from the study of controllable experimental situations. The work began when Medawar's group achieved tolerance to foreign skin by the development of neonatal chimeras and it has been extended to as wide a variety as possible of ways by which an animal can be rendered unresponsive to an antigenic stimulus that would be effective in a normal animal. Particularly since the recognition of the diversity of immunocytes and the interaction of the T and B systems, an immense amount of information has been obtained. As in every other field of immunology, interpretation has lagged behind the accumulation of facts.

For many years I have looked on tolerance as representing a deficiency or absence of immunocytes that can react with the antigenic determinant concerned, and accounted for this by the general statement that the presence of antigen will under appropriate conditions destroy physically or functionally immunocytes bearing an immune pattern with which it can unite. Functional elimination, however, is a phrase which can have many meanings. It is now well established, for example, by Ada, that an animal rendered tolerant to antigen *X* may contain cells capable of taking up labelled *X* in numbers not much inferior to those found in normal animals. Such cells are assumed to be B-lymphocytes and the possibility arises at once that, for these to be stimulated to proliferate, interaction with antigen-reactive T-cells is necessary. Since tolerance or paralysis can involve immune functions mediated by T- and B-type immonocytes, one must assume that on occasion destruction of *X*-reactive T-cells would be adequate to induce tolerance to *X* in the sense of failure of antibody production, even though B-cells reacting with *X* were neither damaged in the process nor stimulated to proliferate. Equally, however, it has been well established under other circumstances that tolerance can be produced inhibiting antibody production without T-cells being involved.

One must agree with Dresser and Mitchison that there is no positive experimental proof that physical destruction of immunocytes is the basis of tolerance and paralysis. Equally, however, no one has disproved such a contention and there have been several demonstrations that if immunocytes of a defined character are specifically removed or destroyed the experimental system behaves as one from a tolerant or paralysed animal would behave. Evidence, admittedly still indirect, in favour of destruction may be deduced from the need for

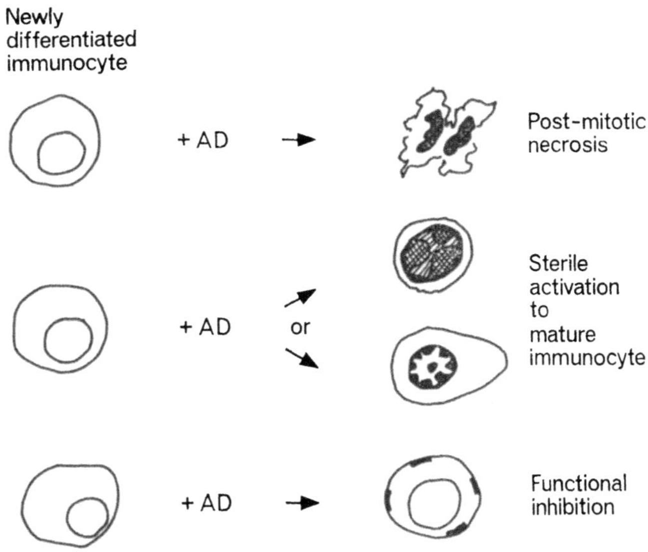

FIG. 12. Possible ways by which natural tolerance develops. In each case there can be no clonal expansion of the cell line.

complement to be present if an antigen is to produce tolerance or paralysis. I shall therefore continue to adopt the same essential approach as I used in the first formulation of clonal selection theory: that contact with antigen at an early stage in the differentiation of immunocytes has a high probability of destroying the cells that can react with it. In *Cellular Immunology* I have qualified this simple approach to bring quantitative factors into the picture, but I have in no sense abandoned the basic hypothesis. There is direct evidence that lymphoblasts, in situations where cell-based immunological reactions are occurring, frequently suffer morphological death, often in the immediate post-mitotic phase. Experimental evidence of specific death by antigen contact may well never be obtainable. All the evidence we have is functional and there are two other possibilities by which, without physical destruction, the observed findings could be produced. The cell could be forced into sterile activation, becoming an antibody-producing plasma cell without capacity for proliferation. *One* antibody-producing cell is irrelevant, even in a mouse. Alternatively, some simpler type of inhibition without activation could be considered which might even still allow the presence of receptors on the cell surface. However, having regard to what we know of the general aspects of cellular function, elimination by actual cellular death and removal by autolysis and phagocytosis seems likely to be the commonest mechanism. After all, this is what happens when in the course of differentiation and metamorphosis special populations of cells become redundant. There is general agreement that recovery from immune paralysis results predominantly by recruitment of new immunocytes. I know of no positive evidence that cells can be rendered immunologically inert and subsequently revived to full activity. A number of claims to show that something of the sort occurs all seem to have alternative explanations.

The elimination of unneeded immunocytes

With this background, our concept of tolerance and paralysis can be developed on the basis of my original formulation (Burnet, 1959) to a form which is in general conformity with the findings reviewed by Dresser and Mitchison (1968). The essence of differentiation either to T- or B-immunocyte is the synthesis of antibody in the form of a cell membrane receptor. On the T-cell the receptor is equivalent to a monomeric form of IgM, i.e. it possesses the characteristic κ and μ antigens but has a molecular weight in the neighbourhood of 180,000 instead of the 900,000 of the standard pentameric form. The early forms of B-cells probably also carry IgM receptors, but in larger numbers and of pentamer type. In addition, there is evidence of continuing synthesis and liberation of such antibody receptors. A proportion of such cells can, under appropriate circumstances, switch to IgG production. Whether immunocytes of clones which will eventually produce IgA, IgD, or IgE are first differentiated with IgM receptors is not known.

For obvious technical reasons nearly all the relevant experiments have been concerned with the conditions under which antibody is produced, usually in mice, sometimes in rabbits. There is enough evidence to indicate that similar principles hold for the production of sensitization or desensitization to T-immune responses. There are, however, several important differences which emerge with suitable experimental material. The specificity of the T-cell receptors is much less restricted, as judged by DH reactions, than those of B-cells judged by antibody. The molecular basis of this difference is unknown. Further, there are well-established examples in which tolerance in the B system can be associated with full sensitization to the same antigen in the T system. In many situations, however, the response of both systems to a single antigenic determinant can be eliminated together, particularly when tolerance is induced in the neonatal animal.

Tolerance or paralysis develops, according to Dresser and Mitchison, whenever even small amounts of antigen can persist for significant periods without provoking an immune response. Once an immune response has been provoked, relatively large amounts of antigen are needed to induce paralysis. Any actual experiment is bound to be complicated by secondary factors, but, broadly speaking, one can say:

1. That immunocytes that have just undergone differentiation are relatively susceptible to destruction by antigen.

2. That immunocytes in foetal and very young animals can only rarely react to proliferate and produce antibody.

3. That antigen associated with macrophages, in particular with the dendritic phagocytic cells (DPC) of lymphoid tissue, is, other things being equal, likely to provoke a positive immune response, while free antigen is likely to induce cell destruction, and tolerance.

4. Once significant numbers of B-immunocytes and a certain amount of antibody have been produced, further small amounts of antigen will be selectively taken up by DPC and act as a secondary stimulus to proliferation and antibody production. When large amounts of a soluble antigen are injected intravenously in an immunized animal, it may be possible for an excess of antigen to persist at a level which is destructive to all corresponding immunocytes, so inducing complete immune paralysis.

Intrinsic tolerance

On the general basis for immunological reactivity that we have adopted there is more than one way by which the body can ensure that damaging immune reactions with its own cells and tissues do not occur.

1. It may be genetically impossible for immune patterns to be produced which can react significantly with some molecular configurations.

On general grounds one can feel certain that there are many organic configurations which are non-antigenic because there is no combining site that can be produced by the interaction of two 'variable' peptide chains which will react with them. For other configurations there may be no categorical inability to produce an appropriate combining site but a very low probability of its emergence.

For such 'poor' antigens, minor genetic differences may be such that animal *A* can never produce such an antibody, while animal *B* can do so under appropriate circumstances. From another angle it is by no means inconceivable that on a living cell surface there are macromolecules which present no antigenic aspects in the intact animal but which, when disorganized by homogenization, could be antigenic even in the autologous animal. There are experiments which are compatible with such an interpretation but none in which it has been shown that this is the only reasonable interpretation.

2. Potential antigens on cell surfaces or becoming accessible in the course of normal physiological processes are incapable of making immunogenic contact with immunocyte receptors.

This is closely related to (1) but would also cover such possibilities as shielding of antigenic determinants by sialic acid-containing mucoids or any other structural component.

3. Potential antigens in cells are so situated that under all normal conditions they have no contact with immunocytes.

Organ-specific potential antigens in solid organs represent the most important group. It is implicit here that small amounts of such inaccessible antigens must on many occasions escape into the circulation. Such amounts are insufficient to stimulate a T-immune response.

4. Any cells carrying immune patterns reactive with accessible body antigens are destroyed at an early stage after their differentiation to immunocytes.

This is the central approach to tolerance and will be extensively discussed later.

One can almost summarize all four points by saying that intrinsic tolerance demands that there be only minimal numbers of immunocytes which can react with body antigens, and minimal 'exposure' of potential antigens that are not necessarily always exposed.

It is both teleologically reasonable and in line with the experimental findings to assume that elimination of immunocytes bearing immune receptors that react with 'self' antigenic determinants should take place predominantly with cells which had only recently differentiated from stem cells. Such cells will differ in a number of ways from mature immunocytes, including the strictness of the specificity of their immune receptors. However, as in all immunological discussion, there is nothing predetermined about the 'goodness of fit' or affinity between antigenic determinant and cell receptor. Union, when it occurs, will influence the immunocyte in ways depending on its relative maturity and other factors which are better considered in relation to pharmacological aspects of the immune response.

In broad terms, if it is a B-immunocyte it may be lethally damaged, it may be stimulated to proliferate as a memory cell, it may initiate an active clone of plasma cells, or it may undergo a terminal (sterile) differentiation to a plasma cell. The possibility too is still open that union of antigenic determinant with B-cell receptor may have no stimulatory effect at all, either because an insufficient number of receptors are concerned or for some other reason. The observed changes in number of antibody-producing cells or in the level of circulating antibody, and hence the degree of tolerance or non-responsiveness, will depend on the proportion of reactive cells undergoing each type of reaction.

If a T-cell is involved, we have the alternatives of destruction or sub-lethal damage, both with the liberation of pharmacologically active agents, lymphokines, proliferation as memory cells, and possibly some other changes of which mast cell transformation is probably most worth consideration. Which type of change will result depends on a number of parameters, of which those most relevant in the present context are: (1) the physiological state and degree of maturity of the cell; (2) the concentration of the reacting antigenic determinant; and (3) the affinity of union. The influence of (2) and (3) could probably be combined and represented as a complex function which might take the form of the proportion of cell receptors united to antigenic determinant at any given instant. As will be discussed later, it is probably premature to assume that intensity of stimulation is a simple function of the proportion of cell receptors occupied. All we can be sure of is that there are rules which determine changes in the type of cell response in relation to the intensity of antigenic stimulation.

This type of quantitative approach to antigen-receptor interactions is basic to the understanding of partial tolerance, the production of auto-antibodies in experimental animals and many of the phenomena of auto-immune disease in man. In the normal healthy animal it ensures that any immunocytes (B or T) which emerge on differentiation with an immune receptor which has a significant degree of reactivity for any widely distributed and accessible antigenic determinant within the body will be completely and rapidly eliminated.

We can assume that differentiation takes place in lymphoid tissue in the broadest sense, including thymus and bone marrow, i.e. in a region where lymphoid cells are actively proliferating and where other cells are dying and being autolysed. In such an environment an extremely wide range of potential antigenic determinants will be immediately accessible, including all the surface antigens of mononuclear cells of various type and red cells, all the constituents of plasma and lymph, and a wide variety of intracellular components including nuclear fragments, histones, and nucleic acids. All histocompatibility antigens, all red cell antigens and an immense range of peptide and nucleotide configurations must be included in the accessible antigens. The rule will hold that no recently differentiated B- or T-immunocyte will survive which reacts significantly with any of these thousands of potential antigens. Despite the postulated destruction of cells with all these immune patterns, there are still large numbers which are not significantly affected by any and so are available for eventual reaction with some foreign antigenic determinant.

There will, however, always be borderline situations. A cell may only just fail to be eliminated by the available concentration of a genuine accessible self-antigen X. If now X is injected in large amount with adjuvant into such an animal, it is highly probable that a detectable concentration of low-affinity antibody against X will be produced. A failure of natural tolerance can then be reported. Similarly, if there are two or more ways of assaying anti-X and one is more sensitive (in detecting low-affinity antibody) than the other, tolerance may be demonstrated by one method, not by the other.

Partial tolerance and related topics

Accepting the situation that in the healthy animal there are no immunocytes significantly reactive against any accessible antigenic determinants and that this is the basis for the observed failure to produce antibody against autologous constituents of the body, there is still scope for complication. As will be discussed later, there are several ways by which a genetically normal animal can be made to produce antibody against a self-antigen: a fact highly relevant to the understanding of auto-immune disease.

In dealing with auto-immune disease we are necessarily concerned

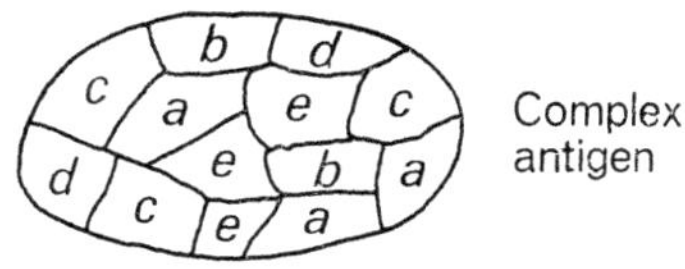

Normal antibody	*A*	*B*	*C*	*D*	*E*
Acquired tolerance	–	–	–	–	–
Recovery	–	–	*C*	–	–
↓	–	–	*C*	–	*E*
	–	*B*	*C*	–	*E*
	A	*B*	*C*	–	*E*

FIG. 13. Piecemeal recovery of immune competence. Normal antibody includes the produce of clones against all the foreign antigenic determinants in a complex antigen. With tolerance, none of the antibodies are produced on challenge with antigen. With the progressive lapse of time, challenge gives responses of the general type shown. *a*, *b*, *c*, etc. = antigenic determinants. *A*, *B*, *C*, etc. = the corresponding antibodies.

with highly complex cellular antigens, almost certainly including a number of different antigenic determinants. This holds too for any standard protein antigen, a foreign serum albumin for example. An instructive example of partial tolerance, almost certainly due to multiplicity of antigenic determinants, is found in the process by which an animal rendered non-responsive by neonatal injection of a foreign serum albumin becomes again responsive. Humphrey (1964) studied this in some detail in rabbits given a single injection of human serum albumin (HSA) immediately after birth. The primary test for recovery of immune capacity was the time at which an immune elimination response developed. This varied greatly from one animal to another. In some there was no response till long after all antigen must have been removed from the body and, in all, the early responses were poor in quality with antibody that was non-precipitating and low in avidity. Humphrey summarized his results by saying that paralysis was a function of whole antigenic molecules, i.e. of all their antigenic determinants, but that the 'capacity to respond returns piecemeal in respect to different parts of the antigenic mosaic'.

A more specific interpretation would be to say that the large injection of HSA at birth resulted in the annihilation of all immunocytes sufficiently reactive with any of the antigenic determinants of the HSA molecule, and a continued elimination of any that appeared while adequate amounts of the foreign antigen remained in circulation. In the older animals, newly emerged immunocytes appear more slowly than in the perinatal period and there are only stochastic regularities in the lag before reactive immunocytes which can develop detectable clones appear. What cannot happen is that a balanced selection of new immune patterns to react with all HSA antigenic determinants should appear simultaneously and allow the full manifestation of all the reactions given by a standard anti-HSA serum.

The special role of T-immunocytes in tolerance

As soon as we begin to contemplate the situation when both T- and B-immunocytes are concerned in the response which interests the investigator, many possibilities of complication and misunderstanding become evident. Miller has recently pointed out that in the mice he works with tolerance to an antigen like a foreign gammaglobulin might mean no more than failure of T-immunocytes to participate. Perfectly normal B-immunocytes could still be available.

There is much to be said for this hypothesis provided we retain the qualification that what is the rule for the CBA mouse may be replaced by something widely different for sheep or man. It must be remembered that the classic concepts of acquired immunological tolerance have been developed in relation to transplants of skin homografts in mice. To interpret the standard results in that field, the simplest and most likely hypothesis is that tolerance results from contact of 'new-born', i.e. newly differentiated, T-immunocytes with specific antigen almost certainly on the surface of foreign chimeric cells or carried passively by some of the animal's own circulating cells. The union of antigen and receptor provides a stimulus to the cell, which is either directly destructive or provokes a sterile activation to an end cell which is functionally equivalent. Tolerance of the T system must axiomatically be present in any tolerant animal, and if all antibodies against normal body components need specifically reactive T-cells to allow antibody production by B-cells, no more is needed.

One can, however, both induce antibody production without help from T-cells and render an animal tolerant with a variety of micro-organismal antigens. The B system can obviously be rendered intrinsically tolerant, but we must be wary that this may be merely an artificial result. Miller's view may be of special importance for auto-immunity if, as seems not unlikely, there are *no* potential antigens in the body which are capable of producing antibody by stimulation of B-immunocytes without T-cell co-operation. It is characteristic of mammalian tissues that, to my knowledge, there are only two body components which are composed of regularly recurring units, each of which could serve as an antigenic determinant. These are collagen and elastin, the two types of structural fibre common to all tissues. Both appear to have the same chemical structure in all species and are only demonstrably antigenic when chemically altered. Every structural component of the body chemically considered will present potential antigenic determinants in spatial relationship to other antigenic determinants. Such relationships will take many forms, but, on occasion, one type of antigenic determinant may be related to others in much the same way that hapten relates to carrier antigenic determinants in the widely studied artificial antigens that have been already referred to. Work in this field may therefore sometimes be relevant to auto-immune phenomena and at a later stage an interpretation of the Wassermann reaction in such terms will be discussed.

For the present, however, one can accept the importance of T-immunocytes without elaborating rather strained analogies between synthetic antigens and the much more complex situation in the body. For any potential antigenic determinant intrinsic to the body or introduced, the result of specific contact with either T- or B-immunocytes will be governed by certain rules. Probably the most that can be said is that there are conditions which will allow the cell to proliferate and produce antibody with a certain probability and other conditions when there is a definite probability that the cells will be eliminated from immunocytic function.

Finally, a little should be said about tolerance as it is manifested in one of the best-studied experimental models using *Salmonella* flagellar protein in the rat. Here the dosage of antigen has a predominant influence in deciding whether a B-cell produces antibody or not. Using flagellin as antigen (one not requiring T-cell interaction) in both *in vivo* and *in vitro* experiments, the following results are established (Nossal and Ada, 1971).

1. *In vivo*, using rats, partial tolerance is produced with fantastically low doses of antigen (low zone tolerance).

2. Then follows a zone of antigen concentration in which proliferation and antibody production is observed both *in vivo* and *in vitro*.

3. With higher doses, tolerance results again both *in vivo* and *in vitro*.

4. *In vitro* addition of small amounts of preformed antibody can allow tolerance to be produced at a concentration which would otherwise be immunogenic.

Mainly because I can see no biological significance for it I am inclined to neglect low zone tolerance as an interesting artifact only. High zone tolerance has the important implication that it represents a potential second line of defence against auto-immune clones. The power of antibody to, as it were, make high zone tolerance possible at a lower level is in all probability due to the power of antibody to concentrate together more antigenic determinants to be focused destructively on a single cell.

Even with flagellin new complications are always appearing. Parish (1971), for instance, has emphasized that delayed hypersensitivity (DH) can be clearly shown with flagellins. So can tolerance at the DH level, but its behaviour is very different from tolerance or paralysis at the antibody level. The most striking finding is that modification of the monomeric flagellin by aceto-acetylation greatly diminishes its immunogenic power to produce antibody, makes it a better tolerogen and increases its capacity to induce cell-mediated immunity (DH). Equally important is the lower specificity of DH and of (antibody) tolerance. There is virtually no cross-reaction between two flagellins from *S. adelaide* and *S. typhimurium*, but there is strong cross-reaction at the DH level and a rat rendered tolerant to *S. adelaide*, as judged by antibody response, is almost equally unresponsive to *S. typhimurium* flagellin.

In adult rats, tolerance produced by aceto-acetylated flagellin is only antibody tolerance; DH is more active, but given to neonatal rats tolerance involves both antibody and cell-mediated immunity.

Summary

In many ways modern work has greatly complicated the theoretical approach to tolerance without as yet allowing any useful application to medicine. No active investigator could possibly accept the following statement, but perhaps from the point of view of developing a good provisional understanding of auto-immunity it may be helpful.

Tolerance represents the absence of the immunocytes or specific combinations of immunocytes necessary for the mounting of an immune response against the antigen in question.

Its natural significance is solely in regard to normal body components, cellular and soluble, and in this area T-immunocytes are always important.

B-immunocytes are concerned primarily with anti-bacterial defence. Tolerance is biologically unwanted, but there must be a feedback control to prevent undue production of a single antibody type.

A secondary involvement of B-immunocytes in immune responses to circulating cells and plasma proteins can develop and is of high importance in some auto-immune diseases.

CHAPTER 5

Pharmacological aspects of immune responses

Unless all our interpretations are wrong, the significant interactions between immunocyte and antigen always involve the stimulation of the cell by contact of antigenic determinant (AD) with a cell surface receptor. In other words AD acts essentially as a drug acts on its appropriate receptor. It may well emerge that neither immunology nor pharmacology has developed sufficiently for any application of pharmacological principles to be helpful in the interpretation of immunological phenomena. Nevertheless, it seems essential at this point to include some account of what seem to be relevant aspects of current pharmacological teaching.

Drug receptors

The first point to be looked at is the nature of drug receptors. In general, following Paton (1970), we can postulate that drug receptors are cell surface molecular configurations, almost certainly proteins, whose physiological function is to serve as a receptor for some hormone or transmitter such as acetylcholine, and to initiate a signal calling on the cell for appropriate functional activity. Corresponding to each such receptor there will be a family of drugs structurally akin to the natural agent and therefore capable of influencing the receptor: either agonists capable of positive stimulation or antagonists which reduce or abolish its sensitivity to physiological or synthetic agonists. It must be kept in mind, of course, that not all the normal transmitters and hormones are known. Allowing for these receptors of still unknown physiological function, Paton expresses the opinion that there may be no more than fifty types of genetically coded receptors.

Most of the evidence for the existence of drug receptors has been more or less indirect and the recent isolation of a receptor protein of known function is therefore important. In the electric tissue of the fish *Torpedo* there are cholinergic receptors which are apparently identical with the acetylcholine receptors of the neuromuscular junctions of vertebrates.

They are present, however, in vastly greater numbers in the electric tissue and this allowed the protein responsible to be obtained. Its isolation followed study of the pharmacological activities of snake venom from the Formosan krait (*Bungarus*). This has been known for some time to block specifically and irreversibly the depolarizing action of acetylcholine at neuromuscular receptors. It has now been shown by Miledi *et al.* (1971) that the purified active component from *Bungarus* venom also binds firmly with the receptor protein when it is free in solution and allows its isolation. They conclude that the acetylcholine receptor is a membrane-bound protein of approximately 80,000 molecular weight. The number of bungarotoxin binding sites appears to be numerically equal to the number of acetylcholinesterase sites, but the receptor protein is quite distinct from the enzyme. The point to be stressed is that this and, by implication, other drug receptors are specifically structured proteins with combining sites which must be broadly similar to the specific receptors of immunocytes.

Paton's rate theory of pharmacological stimulation is that excitation is proportional to the rate of association of the drug with the receptor; if this is associated with a high dissociation rate, the drug will have a high efficacy. When there is firm binding, i.e. low dissociation rate with prolonged occupancy, there will be antagonism to the action of an effective drug of the same series. The interaction of agonists and antagonists is often highly complex. In many instances the initial action of the agonist is to desensitize the receptor for a period and to change its affinity for antagonists and partial agonists. Most such work has been done purely at the pharmacological level and the molecular nature of the drug-receptor interaction is unknown.

An important recent advance is the recognition that many types of receptor, particularly those specific for peptide and protein hormones, initiate their signal to the cell by activating an enzyme, adenyl cyclase, which converts ATP to cyclic adenosine monophosphate (Cy-AMP) which has been called a common 'second messenger'.

Stimulation of immunocyte (ARC) by antigen

It is not easy to bring these ideas into a useful relationship with immunological phenomena. Nevertheless, it seems to be a logical first approach to regard the antibody-like immune receptor as basically analogous to any drug (hormone)-receptor at the cell membrane. The most obvious field of pharmacological interest is the relationship between antigen concentration, mode of presentation and affinity, on the one hand, and the nature of the response. Under defined conditions with flagellin as antigen, increasing concentration of antigen gives the following sequence of response: low zone tolerance, proliferation of B-immunocytes, high zone tolerance. As Nossal and Ada (1971) put it, the most usual interpretation of this is that 'the cell has some sensing device by which it knows how many surface receptors are occupied by antigen'. For proliferation and antibody production, the number or proportion of receptor sites effectively hit by antigen must be between *a* and *b*. Less than *a* hits results in low zone tolerance, more than *b* in high zone tolerance. In the present state of knowledge, 'hit' is a very imprecise term. We know virtually nothing about how the stimulus is generated by AD-combining site union and in particular as to how stimulus induction is related to the kinetics of reversible union as determined by the affinity constants of the reacting sites involved. The nature of the sensor that interprets the intensity of antigenic impact is therefore quite unknown and there are further complexities. We know that for many types of antibody production interaction between two or more types of cell is required in the presence of antigen. It is equally clear that the effectiveness of a given antigenic determinant as immunogen is greatly dependent on the macromolecule, particle, or cell which carries it. Obviously there is little scope here for the application of simplified pharmacological theories.

There is no doubt about the existence of low zone partial tolerance which, when a 'good' antigen-like flagellin is used, is seen at extraordinarily low doses. One is almost bound to assume that a *single* effective contact of antigenic determinant and receptor may render the cell unavailable to stimulation by other ADs, provided there is a lapse of at least some days before the challenge for tolerance. An armchair speculation which perhaps could suggest some useful experiments is to tabulate a series of possible responses of a reactive immunocyte (a B-type ARC) to successively increasing intensities of stimulation by identical antigenic determinants, starting with a situation where only a single contact takes place.

1. Activation to a sterile antibody-producing cell which at some stage of differentiation becomes insusceptible to further antigenic stimulation.

2. When repeated contacts within shorter periods can occur, we have

activation to proliferation, producing either or both memory cells and a multiplying plasma cell clone.

3. Hyperactivation resulting in post-mitotic death of the stimulated cell.

4. The observation that in some tolerant animals there remain lymphocytes capable of binding the antigen has still not been adequately explained. The possibility could be explored that in cells reacting as (1) the inhibitory process does not result in the disappearance of immune receptors.

Which of these different possibilities will result obviously depends on a variety of factors, including (*a*) the affinity of AD for receptor, (*b*) the concentration of antigen in the cell environment, and (*c*) the time factor. A second series of factors includes (*d*) the mode of presentation of the AD on a cell surface or in solution, (*e*) whether the AD is frequently repeated on the antigen particle or macromolecule, (*f*) the molecular weight of the carrier (cf. Ada's flagellin and the tolerogenic fraction A). Finally, we must also consider (*g*) the physiological state of the cell in relation particularly to its individual age since differentiation, and the age of the animal, and (*h*) the additional complexities which are introduced in those situations where a T-immunocyte must co-operate with the initiator of the antibody-producing line. Clearly there is no scope for a simple statement of cause and effect even at this purely immunological level.

In previous discussions of this general topic I have made use of a diagram to indicate conceptually the relationship of affinity between the reacting active sites and of 'effective concentration' of AD. The latter is a complex parameter including functions of the time the concentration persists, and the mode in which the AD is presented. In Fig. 14 three main areas are shown, with, respectively, no reaction, proliferative stimulation, and lethal stimulation giving high zone tolerance. Very tentatively, a fourth area for low zone tolerance against certain antigens is shown. The figure undoubtedly over-simplifies the situation, in that it takes no account of T- and B-cell interaction or of the different qualities of T- and B-cell stimulation. Studies of the effect of chemical modification of an antigen on its affinity for antibody against the unmodified antigen, on its immunogenicity at B level and its tolerogenic power as tested at both antibody and cell-mediated immunity levels, such as those of Parish mentioned earlier, add still further

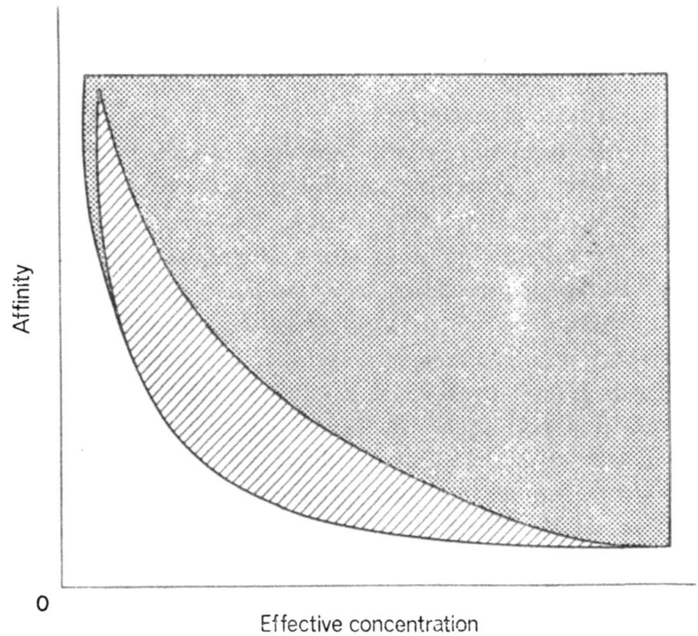

FIG. 14. Tolerance and responsiveness. A graph to indicate how two parameters, affinity of union and effective concentration of antigen, might influence the result of antigen-immunocyte interaction. See text for an account of the difficulties of any such formulation.
Heavy shading = death or inhibition, i.e. tolerance. Light shading = proliferative response. White = no effect.

complexities. It is just possible that the figure could represent a simplified over-all picture of the type of response when the antigenic determinant is a single molecular species and affinity differences concern only the combining sites of immune receptors. One suspects that a figure to represent the 'real' situation would be multidimensional and involve parameters yet to be discovered.

Pharmacologically active agents: lymphokines

Another highly complex situation emerges when we look at what might be called the pharmacological consequences of antigenic stimulation. This may be significant only for T-immunocytes, but there are hints that it must also be associated with the activation of B-cells. So far all this work has been of an exploratory character, the various activities being defined in pharmacological terms; hardly any of the agents liberated and assayed by some biological test have yet been defined at the molecular level. Some pharmacologically active agents previously known and identified, such as histamine and serotonin, are undoubtedly associated with some immune responses, but most of the agents have not been characterized.

Interest in the local and general pathology of immune response was initiated by Koch's discovery of the reaction of the tuberculous guinea-pig to an injection of tuberculin. The crude antigen, tuberculin, or PPD, has no significant effect when injected into a normal guinea-pig, but produces fever, local swelling, and other damaging effects in a tuberculous animal. Ever since, the tuberculin reaction has been the prototype of delayed hypersensitivity and the demonstration that circulating lymphocytes could passively transmit tuberculin sensitization was in a real sense the beginning of cellular immunology. Virtually all studies of the influence of antigen on sensitized cells were initiated with lymphocytes from tuberculous animals or human beings. Later, similar reactions involving other types of antigen were demonstrated. The main phenomena observed when sensitized lymphocytes reacted with the corresponding antigen are: (*a*) a proportion of lymphocytes are transformed to blasts and these then undergo mitosis; (*b*) lymphocytes cytotoxic for target cells liberate a lymphotoxin (LT) which has a destructive effect on the target cell; similar findings are obtained when 'sensitized' lymphocytes are exposed to the specific antigen and when normal lymphocytes are treated with a non-specific mitogen such as PHA; (*c*) a migratory inhibitory factor (MIF), which can prevent the migration of macrophages *in vitro*, is produced under the same circumstances as LT and may be the same material; (*d*) a factor that stimulates macrophages to take up bacteria more effectively (Mackaness) is also liberated. All these phenomena are presumably based on the production of lymphokines.

It is highly probable that lymphocytes may also be induced to produce lymphokines by a cascade effect in the sense that an immunocyte is stimulated by specific antigen to produce lymphokines which, in sufficient concentration, will non-specifically provoke adjacent lymphocytes to produce more lymphokines and so on. Cascade processes of this type are seen in relation to blood clotting, where the obvious dangers are countered by an elaborate series of inhibitors. The evidence for the existence of a cascade effect in the present field comes mainly from the realization that most of the cells observed in a homograft rejection or a typical delayed hypersensitivity reaction are not specifically reactive to the corresponding antigen. Precisely similar results have recently been obtained in regard to localized auto-immune disease of the adrenal or central nervous system produced experimentally in guinea-pigs.

Another suggestion that has been made is that in the vicinity of a source of antigen many non-specific lymphocytes or monocytes may take up antigenic determinants in their cell membrane. Contact with immunocytes specific to the antigen could then initiate stimulation of both cells. It is relevant here that lymphocytes of the rabbit can be stimulated to blast transformation by an antiserum capable of reacting with immunoglobulin determinants functioning as receptors on the cell membrane.

On the whole, lymphocytes are relatively resistant to lymphotoxins, according to Grainger, but this may not necessarily hold for all phases. It is well known that pyknotic nuclei, 'tingible bodies', are characteristic of any region where lymphoid cells are actively multiplying, such as the thymic cortex or germinal centres. There is evidence of a special susceptibility to damage during mitosis. On the other hand, exposure of a mature lymphocyte to a small concentration of LT can increase its resistance to a subsequent larger dose.

Mast cell function

The role of mast cells in immune responses is still undecided. It is undoubted that antigen, possibly in the form of antigen–antibody complex, can under some circumstances cause discharge of granules from mast cells with liberation of histamine. Current interpretation of the classical anaphylactic experiments is that the liberation of histamine, which is central to them all, is from tissue mast cells, basophil leucocytes, and perhaps platelets. Passive anaphylaxis, as in the standard experiment in which a guinea-pig is given serum from a rabbit immunized with a protein antigen P and then reacts, sometimes fatally, to an intravenous injection of P, must depend on cytophilic antibody taken up by guinea-pig cells. The reaction results from the stimulation of cytophilic antibody on the mast cell surface and this is probably also the most acceptable interpretation of active anaphylaxis in the guinea-pig. There are, however, some suggestions favouring the possibility that some (or all?) mast cells may be immunocytes with antibody-like receptors. I have on other occasions drawn attention to the fact that mouse thymocytes can sometimes undergo a massive, apparently autocatalytic change to mast cells and there are sufficient mast cells in relevant tissues to suggest that they play an active part in some immune responses. During the phase of 'self-cure' of an intestinal infestation in the rat with the nematode worm *Nippostrongylus*, there are greatly increased numbers of mast cells in the submucosa of the intestinal villi.

There is general agreement that mast cells are end cells derived from some other form, presumably fibroblast or lymphocyte. There may well be justification for regarding the mast cell as the final form (analogous to the mature plasma cell of the B series) in which the production of pharmacologically active agents characteristic of all T-immunocytes reaches its acme. This is only a speculative hypothesis, but I have found nothing on record that seriously challenges its validity.

These considerations from the pharmacological side must have some relevance to the pathogenesis of auto-immune disease, but much more understanding both of basic immunological processes and of the clinico-pathological aspects of the various diseases currently described as auto-immune will be needed before much logical application of one to the other can be made. Most of the discussion of pathogenesis will necessarily be left for the sections on particular diseases, but there are a number of points of general interest that should be treated in this chapter.

Cellular actions

The most striking histological evidence of auto-immune disease of local organs or tissues is cellular infiltration, most of the cells appearing like lymphocytes but often with monocytes and eosinophils. Mast cells are not recognizable in conventionally stained sections and are probably more numerous than reports indicate. All these cells must obviously have come from the blood, and the first broad problem is how the blood cells enter the appropriate tissue.

There is now general agreement that in the ordinary course of inflammation the capillary endothelium becomes permeable to motile cells by opening up of the junctions between endothelial cells. It is equally accepted that lymphocytes have a specific capacity to pass through the cytoplasm of the endothelial cells of post-capillary venules in lymphoid tissue. In other tissues too this portion of the vascular network is the most permeable, but I have found no statement as to whether such endothelial cells (in general, non-lymphoid tissues) allow cytoplasmic passage to lymphocytes.

The accepted circulation of lymphocytes is that passage from the blood is predominantly via the post-capillary venules into nodal lymphoid tissue, thence to the collecting sinus of the lymph node and eventually by lymphatic channels to thoracic duct and back to the blood. Another fraction must pass into the general tissues of the body, particularly in the intestinal mucosa, and is collected thence by regional lymphatics. In the lymph nodes it joins the other stream returning to the blood.

The standard teaching is that both in experimental auto-immune encephalomyelitis and in localized auto-immune disease, for example, in the adrenals, the pathogenic cells primarily responsible are lymphocytes produced in lymphoid tissue and reaching their site of action via the blood. These primary cells, we must assume, are immunocytes capable of reacting with an AD specific for the 'target cells' of the organ involved. When the lesion actually develops, however, only a very small porportion of *specifically* reactive cells are involved. As in any delayed hypersensitivity reactions, most of the cells are recently produced lymphocytes plus miscellaneous circulating cells, none of which are immunologically specific. When we concentrate, however, on the essential primary cells, it becomes very important to know (*a*) how the cells 'know' when they are passing through the capillaries of the target organ, and (*b*) how they pass from the lumen of the capillary into the substance of the tissue.

The problem takes its clearest form in experimental encephalomyelitis, since here there can be no suggestion that unrecognized local infection or trauma has initiated the process. When the encephalitogenic protein is injected with adjuvant, proliferation of pathogenic immunocytes presumably takes place in the draining lymph node and initially at least there is no existing inflammation in the brain to attract them. There is some evidence (McFarland, 1969) that lymphocytes attach to the vascular endothelium, in experimental auto-immune neuritis, by the uropod process which *may* carry a concentration of receptors. Irrespective of the significance of the uropod, this observation does give support to the *a priori* hypothesis that the capillary endothelium within an organ will frequently carry on its surface antigenic determinants characteristic of the parenchymatous cells of the organ. Once there is a specifically heightened probability that a reactive immunocyte will be attached immunologically to an endothelial cell in the right organ, a self-amplifying system would naturally develop. The first step would probably be for the pharmacologically active agents liberated by the first cell to make the adjacent endothelium more 'sticky' and hence more likely to hold any other specifically reactive immunocyte passing through that capillary. Soon other specific and non-specific cells will be held and the local situation will become basically the same as a delayed hypersensitivity response, a small proportion of specific immunocytes laying down the conditions that allow large numbers of non-specific lymphocytes and monocytes to enter the tissue at such points.

It is probably an essential characteristic of a local auto-immune process to be self-amplifying once a certain threshold of damage has been achieved. On the afferent side more antigen will be passing to the draining lymph nodes, probably largely on the surface of lymphocytes and monocytes, and more cells of the pathogenic clone engendered there. On the efferent limb the local inflammation with increased capillary permeability will both increase the available concentration of organ antigen on local vascular endothelium and make entry easier for both specifically tuned and non-specific cells. In some organs too an occasional immunocyte will find the conditions appropriate to proliferate locally and found a germinal centre. There are still doubts as to whether a germinal centre is a single clone or provides a site where cells of other clones can proliferate as well. Parenthetically, the major new experimental technique most urgently needed to understand auto-immune disease is a means of isolating and cloning *in vitro* the cells proliferating in the germinal centres that one finds in a thyroid from Hashimoto's disease, in the thymus of myasthenia gravis, or in the salivary glands of Sjögren's disease. If we could define the antigenic determinant responsible in each case, we should be at the beginning of a real understanding of localized auto-immune disease.

Antigen–antibody complexes

The second topic that requires some preliminary discussion is the pathogenic attributes of antigen–antibody complexes. The classic experiments are those of Dixon and his collaborators using repeated large intravenous doses of bovine serum albumin in rabbits. The rabbits varied considerably in their immune responses. Some produced no antibody and showed no symptoms referable to the kidneys; some produced antibody effectively, in amount more than capable of combining with the circulating bovine serum albumin, and these showed no more than transient proteinuria. A final group produced antibody in more or less equivalent amount so that for a substantial period soluble antigen–antibody complexes were circulating. Such animals showed severe glomerulonephritis with proteinuria and raised blood nitrogen. The histological sign of this condition was an accumulation of immunoglobulin-containing material on the glomerular basement membrane. Largely as a result of this work it has become usual to equate this type of basement membrane thickening, as seen, for instance, in the lupus nephritis of SLE patients or in the NZB mice, to the presence of circulating antigen–antibody complexes.

In somewhat similar fashion to the role of specifically pathogenic immunocytes in experimental auto-immune encephalomyelitis, the toxicity of the antigen–antibody complex with attached complement components opens the way for other components of the circulating plasma. In the NZB and NZB×NZW mice, albumin and fibrin were also present in the basement membrane thickenings.

Antigen–antibody soluble complex is probably toxic to any cell it enters and in addition to its effect on the kidney it is also blamed for arteritis and other forms of vasculitis, such as that seen in SLE.

Conclusion

In concluding this summary of those aspects of modern cytology and immunology which seem to be relevant to auto-immune disease, it is hard to avoid leaving an impression of the bewildering complexity of the body's functioning. We are moving in a region too complex to allow the application of a strictly biochemical molecular approach but still far from being susceptible to the commonsense large-scale approach to understanding functions like voluntary movement, digestion, or sense physiology. In almost every field studied at the cytological level the early simple statements about cellular functions have become inadequate. Every new investigation seems to uncover new complexities in the micro- and submicrostructures of the cell. In particular, new interactions dealing with the functional control of the cell are constantly being recognized: genetic control via the genome of the differentiated cell itself and responses to the constant flood of information from its bodily environment via nerve paths and hormonal substances either circulating in the blood or conveying information from adjacent cells.

From the very nature of the experimental method, most investigators must focus only on one facet of such systems. Reading between the lines of many reports one senses a growing sense of futility amongst investigations dealing with the cellular aspects of immunity, inflammation, and repair as studied in conventional preparations. There is a very evident move in the laboratories to get away completely from the too-complex realities of the functioning organism, to model *in vitro* systems in which the normal physiologically necessary controls and interactions of the rest of the body have been eliminated. Most such systems employ some form of cell culture, and so long as the right strain of cell is kept constant (usually by using replicate samples from a large stock stored in liquid nitrogen) and all significant reagents are chemically defined, can be relied on to produce analysable and reproducible results. Unfortunately each such manipulable system is a very incomplete model of the reality that we are nominally seeking to understand. In principle perhaps thousands of such experimental models should in due course allow a 'spin-off' of useful ideas for the better understanding of immunological theory or of the pathogenesis of auto-immune disease.

As yet we are only at the very earliest stage of handling cell cultures of immunocytes and it may be a long time before anyone can be sure he has a pure clone of, shall we say, auto-immunocytes responsible for human auto-immune haemolytic anaemia. Even when this stage has been reached, it is probably unrealistic to expect much help at the clinical and therapeutic level from the cell culture approach. Nowadays, however, it is implicitly accepted that there is an intrinsic justification for creative work in science (even in the conventional fields of medical research) and no need always to be looking over one's shoulder for 'practical applications'. The operational approach in the laboratories is undoutedly that biomedical research will concentrate increasingly on appropriate model systems and exploit them systematically. There is a very relevant precedent in the way that the model system of two old laboratory strains of *Escherichia coli* and two or three bacterial viruses allowed the biochemists to create almost the whole structure of molecular biology. It is immaterial that virtually nothing from molecular biology has yet been applied in medical care. Its achievements must have lifted up the heart of anyone trying to understand his own area of biological scholarship just as the discoveries of quasars and pulsars and the age of the moon rock has excited all of us with any interest in the universe. Even if they are 'useless', they are none the less supreme achievements of the human mind.

I have no doubt that the next generation will create, out of work on model systems of cultured cells, something as significant almost as the double helix or the genetic code. Perhaps it will be concerned with the molecular structure and basic functions of the informational proteins of the cell membrane. Even if only a lesser degree of generalization is attained, there will be exhilaration for future immuno-pathologists in the results of cloning and defining the functional abnormalities in the immunocytes responsible for auto-immune disease and the various malignant and semi-malignant processes: without worrying at all whether the information will have any bearing on the handling of the corresponding diseases in man.

CHAPTER 6

Infection and auto-immunity

Chronic disease in man, like the general process of ageing, may usually depend on changes intrinsic to the body, but the environment can never be forgotten. Auto-immune manifestations may be modified by cold and exposure, by microbial infection, and by psychosocial factors. In recent years there have been many indications that, in one way or another, infection can have an important influence in modifying or even initiating auto-immune disease.

Closely related is the other recently recognized quality that, in many virus diseases, symptoms and histopathological changes depend not so much on damage to cells by the virus as on the immunological reactions to the infection. This is probably almost equally true for many chronic diseases including tuberculosis, leprosy (especially the lepromatous type), and syphilis. These phenomena are of great intrinsic interest, but in addition they have had an important influence on general thinking about auto-immune disease that justifies brief discussion. This will, however, be limited to examples from viral disease except for brief attention to the significance of auto-antibody production in syphilis.

Symptoms from immune response in viral disease

At the experimental level, the virus disease, chronic lymphocytic choriomeningitis of mice, was the earliest, and is still the best studied, example. The disease was first recognized by the occurrence of severe febrile disease in a laboratory worker in the Rockefeller Institute in 1935. The virus isolated from him was eventually found to be persistently present in one of the Institute mouse stocks. Its behaviour in such an infected colony was studied by Shope and Traub, who uncovered what at that time was a unique situation. Adult mice contained virus in all organs and the young were born congenitally infected. None showed any sign of illness and were unaffected by injection of virus intracerebrally or by any other route. The virus could in fact only be detected by using mice from other colonies that had never become infected. Intracerebral injection in such mice produced lethal disease, transmissible serially like any other infection by a neurotropic virus. Mice killed with fully developed symptoms showed extensive lymphocytic infiltration around the cerebral capillaries and venules. Infection of new-born mice did not cause symptoms and they developed a persisting, symptomless infection. Further, grown animals show no symptoms if immediately after inoculation they are treated by X-irradiation or cortisone in dose adequate to prevent a lymphocytic response. Young adult mice that have been neonatally thymectomized also fail to show symptoms.

The accepted interpretation of these phenomena is that intrinsically the virus is a temperate one which can proliferate in a wide variety of cells without causing significant damage. If it enters the embryo *in utero* or is injected into the neonatal animal, sufficient antigen is produced to render the animal tolerant as far as the T-immune system is concerned. There is no proliferation of T-immunocytes and no response to the infection. In a previously uninfected mature animal, however, the proliferation of virus liberates antigen which stimulates T-immunocyte proliferation and what is essentially a delayed hypersensitivity reaction in the infected brain and meninges. It is this reaction which produces symptoms and death.

Changes in the B system in the persisting tolerated infections are not so well established. Antibody is difficult to detect by standard methods, but there is now convincing evidence that the kidney lesions commonly found in these mice as they grow older are due to the deposition of antigen–antibody complexes in the glomeruli and that the antigen concerned is specific for LCM virus. It may be important that this type of renal disease is seen only in certain strains of mice.

Measles is the best known of human infectious diseases and there have been abundant opportunities to observe its behaviour in children with many different types of immunological deficiency. The fact that measles shows a normal course and subsequent firm immunity in children with congenital agammaglobulinaemia (i.e. with no functioning B system) has already been discussed. From this and much other evidence it seems clear that the rash and other symptoms of measles essentially represent a cell-mediated T-type response to infection by a virus which would otherwise produce either no symptoms or a subacute, usually fatal, giant cell pneumonia with a rash.

Another important example concerns Jennerian vaccination against smallpox. Again, much can be learnt from unforeseen 'experiments of nature' in which a child with some known or as yet unsuspected immunological anomaly is vaccinated. Most children with agammaglobulinaemia respond normally to vaccination. They lack a B system but T responses are unchanged. In deficiencies involving the T system, generalized and indolently spreading infection may occur after vaccination and is usually fatal. Treatment with immune gammaglobulin has no effect on the condition.

On the experimental side it is possible to render neonatal rabbits immunologically unresponsive by injection of large amounts of inactivated vaccinia virus. For several months at least these rabbits produce no antibody and show no skin reaction to vaccinia virus antigens. If such tolerant animals are tested with active virus in the skin, no more than a minimal lesion appears. There is very little multiplication at the site of injection, but the virus spreads freely through the body and most of the rabbits die. By contrast, when this is done in normal non-tolerant young rabbits, there is a typical local lesion going through the stages of macule, papule, vesicle, and ulcer, with free proliferation of virus and a zone of surrounding inflammation. None of the rabbits show generalization or die. Possibly the most important point to be emphasized here is that when there is an effective T response the virus is localized but can proliferate freely. With some viruses, such as that of vesicular stomatitis, proliferation cannot occur in normal human lymphocytes, but it can when these have been stimulated to blast transformation. This has in fact been made the basis for a method of assaying the extent to which transformation by an antigen occurs in given lymphocyte populations.

It may be necessary to bear in mind that the occurrence of a localized immune or auto-immune response may make available a nidus for viral multiplication that would not otherwise occur, much in the way that certain human tumours tend to 'attract' EB virus. The frequent occurrence of a low-grade virus or a mycoplasma in a given lesion is by no means decisive evidence that it is etiologically responsible for the condition.

Rheumatic fever

Rheumatic fever is never classed as an auto-immune disease. It has a well-defined etiology (streptococcal infection in the tonsillar region) and recurrence after a first attack can be avoided with considerable certainty by regular prophylactic use of penicillin. Nevertheless, there is a genetic predisposition to the disease and all pathologists are agreed that there are no streptococci multiplying in the joint lesions of the acute initial stage or in the myocardial or valvular lesions of any subsequent heart involvement. It is known that there are shared antigenic determinants in the surface components of haemolytic streptococci of group A and in myocardial tissue. The corresponding antibodies recognized as reacting with cardiac muscle by immunofluorescent techniques are much commoner in rheumatic fever patients than in those with uncomplicated streptococcal pharyngitis. This holds too for anti-streptolysin-O and other antibodies against streptococcal products.

It is not easy to incorporate these aspects into a general account of the pathogenesis of what is a highly variable disease. In attempting to do so I shall use basically the same approach as in a previous account (Burnet, 1969) brought up to date at one or two points. The genetic predisposition of perhaps 2–3 per cent of persons of European descent appears to depend on their capacity to produce an exceptionally vigorous immune response. It is probably significant that rheumatic fever is the only important disease with a peak of incidence and mortality between the ages of 6 and 13 years: a time which, of all the 'ages of man', is otherwise the least vulnerable to disease.

A subacutely inflamed tonsil heavily infected with streptococci has many resemblances to the granuloma produced when an antigen is injected experimentally with Freund's complete adjuvant. In the predisposed individual this provides opportunity for the expansion of any immunocyte lines capable of reaction with streptococcal antigenic determinants, with the emergence, as a result, of clones of T-immunocytes as well as of a wide range of antibody-producing clones.

For both B and T responses the antigenic determinant that is recognized by immunofluorescent reaction on cardiac muscle is probably the most important. The cardiac antigen appears to be normally inaccessible in the sense that normal individuals show no antibody, but a high proportion of persons subjected to open heart surgery and a smaller group of patients with acute cardiac infarction do develop the antibody after the episode of cardiac damage. It is indicative of the importance of the antibody that Kaplan found the cardiac muscle of five children dying of hyperacute rheumatic carditis heavily coated with immunoglobulin. There seems to be a probability that such accumulation of antibody may have been preceded and made possible by the entry of 'aggressive' T-immunocytes of similar specificity.

There is no similar evidence of a specific antigen being present in joint synovia, but the possibility is not excluded. Joints are characteristically involved in serum sickness and in other situations where circulating antigen–antibody complexes are concerned. In a subacutely infected tonsil there are doubtless opportunities for a variety of streptococcal products and fragments to enter lymph and blood circulations and for antigen–antibody complexes to be circulating. They will lodge in many places, but symptomatic evidence of lodgement will be most conspicuous in the joints. The well-known migratory character of the joint involvement presumably means that, once a small local lesion is initiated in a joint, local inflammation makes it easier for further pathogenic material to lodge or to become more accessible in adjacent parts of the joint.

In many ways it would be legitimate to speak of rheumatic carditis as an auto-immune disease in which the streptococcal antigen is an effective stimulant for the production of antibody and T-immunocytes reactive with an 'inaccessible' myocardial antigen.

The Wassermann reaction

It has been evident ever since the Wassermann antigen was first prepared from normal livers that most of the serological tests for syphilis were detecting auto-antibodies. The position became even more challenging when it was recognized that biological false positive reactions to complement fixation or precipitin tests for syphilis were commonly seen in association with SLE and sometimes with other auto-immune diseases.

The standard antigen in Wassermann reactions (WR) or Kahn tests is a diphospholipid, cardiolipin (CL), which is a mitochondrial constituent of all tissue cells. A current interpretation (Wright *et al.*, 1970) is that the phospholipid hapten is also present as a component of *Treponema pallida*, but bound, of course, to a different carrier protein. This is perhaps the most important example in support of the view mentioned earlier that there may be many potential B antigenic determinants in the body which are completely non-immunogenic because there is full intrinsic tolerance of the T system to all the proteins these determinants are associated with. By implication, the antigen CL-carrier requires an association of appropriately reactive B- and T-immunocytes if antibody is to be produced. In syphilis at least two anti-treponemal antibodies are produced and there is evidence of T-type responses so that there is *a priori* justification for the concept that CL-treponema antigen could produce an antibody when CL-body protein will not. On the whole this interpretation fits well with the facts that a positive WR is usually not associated with any symptoms or signs of auto-immune disease. It is equally in accord with the finding that biological false positive WRs are nearly always in persons with other signs of auto-immune disease.

Here we have a first-rate example of the two ways in which an auto-antibody can appear, both depending on the predominant role of carrier protein in relation to tolerance. In the first, the indications are strong that the capacity of *T. pallida* to synthesize or incorporate into its structure the hapten cardiolipin allows the production of anti-hapten, which could not occur in the normal individual. In the person predisposed to auto-immune disease, the natural composite antigen(s), self protein-cardiolipin, is auto-immunogenic because of the existence of T-immunocytes, capable as a result of genetic and/or somatic genetic anomaly of interacting with the self component which serves as carrier.

Pathogenesis of slow virus infections

The possibility that chronic infection with slow viruses may be concerned in the etiology of auto-immune disease has been widely canvassed in recent years. The experimental and observational basis for this opinion comes from work on Aleutian disease of mink and haemolytic anaemia in NZB mice. Another quite distinct approach has been via scrapie in sheep and kuru, an exotic disease of the indigenes of part of the New Guinea Highlands. None of these conditions are particularly well known and a brief description of each, with special relevance to its 'auto-immune' and virological aspects, seems necessary.

Aleutian mink disease is observed almost exclusively in two types of colour mutants (Aleutian and Sapphire) in which a recessive gene *a* is present in double dose. The principal characteristics of the disease are hypergammaglobulinaemia, excessive plasma cells, periarteritis, and chronic kidney disease. It is possible to obtain *aa* mink without the disease and transfer it to them by injection of cell-free material from an affected mink. The transmissible agent has not been grown in tissue culture and has an exceptional resistance to formalin. Apparently present in all *aa* mink is a genetic anomaly of the leucocytes analogous to the human Chediak–Higashi syndrome which is associated with giant granules in the polymorphonuclear leucocytes and an undue susceptibility to infection.

The NZB mouse disease is described in a later section. The evidence that its inherited characteristic of developing auto-immune haemolytic anaemia some time after six months of age is due to a vertically transmitted virus is very slender. Electron-microscopic evidence of virus particles has been found in some stocks of the strain and the reticulum cell tumours common in older mice resemble tumours produced by oncogenic viruses in other mouse strains.

Kuru, scrapie, and Creutzfeld–Jakob disease need to be considered together, along with ataxia-telangiectasia and cerebellar degeneration associated with malignant disease. All are characterized by progressive degeneration of cerebellar function with loss of Purkinje cells. From the first three a transmissible agent has produced similar disease in experimental animals.

Scrapie is a disease of sheep, with a clear limitation to animals of a double recessive *ss* genotype and showing first syptoms after two years of age. Affected animals have sensory disturbances, probably based on lesions in the thalamic region; they apparently produce an intolerable itch, causing the sheep to rub themselves frantically against any suitable object: hence the name scrapie. In addition, cerebellar-type ataxia develops and progresses. Brain material from a sheep with typical symptoms given by intracerebral injection will convey a similar disease to sheep, goats, or mice, with an incubation period of three to eighteen months. The transmissible agent is highly resistant to heat and formalin and has never been visualized in electron-micrographs.

According to current interpretations, kuru results (or resulted, for it is now a vanishing disease) from ritual consumption by cannibals of partially cooked brain from a previous victim of the disease. In the period 1958–62, it was by far the commonest cause of death in adult women in an isolated area of the Eastern Highlands of New Guinea. It was seen in females from 7 to 40 or 50 and in males during childhood but very rarely in adult men. Basically, the disease is a rapidly progressive cerebellar degeneration with destruction of Purkinje cells and usually dense astrocytosis. From the onset of symptoms to death the course of the disease is inexorably progressive, killing usually in between six and twelve months. Brain from a victim produces similar symptoms and pathological changes when inoculated intracerebrally in chimpanzees. The incubation period is over a year. More recently, infection has also been produced in spider monkeys.

Creutzfeldt–Jakob disease is a rare pre-senile encephalopathy, some cases of which show a spongy degeneration of cortical and cerebellar cells not unlike what is seen in kuru, especially in experimentally inoculated chimpanzees. Biopsy materials from three such patients have now produced in chimpanzees a basically similar disease with an incubation period of about thirteen months.

Finally, we have the genetic disease of children, ataxia-telangiectasia, in which cerebellar degeneration is combined with conspicuous superficial blood vessels on conjunctiva and facial skin and with moderately severe 'mixed' immunological deficiency involving mainly the T system. Malignant tumours of lymphoid tissue are particularly common in these patients.

Cerebellar degeneration, histologically and clinically very similar to kuru, is one of the rarer types of central or peripheral nervous disease associated with malignancy that Lord Brain discussed extensively. Neither in these cases nor in children with ataxia-telangiectasia have attempts to isolate viruses been recorded.

None of the seven human or animal diseases that have been enumerated have been fully elucidated. Aleutian mink disease is said by one experienced group of workers to occur only in mink with a genetic anomaly associated with diminished immune responses and it is by no means clear that the same infectious agent was concerned in all transmission experiments. One must conclude that it is hardly relevant to any human aspect of auto-immune disease.

The NZB and NZB/W mice show conditions with a real relevance to human auto-immune haemolytic anaemia and SLE respectively, as will be elaborated later. Any part played by a type C oncogenic virus as found in certain stocks is not proven.

The scrapie–kuru group is in a wholly different category. The scrapie transmissible agent may be a virus: defined as a self-replicating entity with an RNA or DNA genome coding for a small number of proteins but making use of the host's metabolic machinery; but the present evidence suggests that it is a transmissible agent of some quite different character. None of the suggested alternatives have any positive findings to support them. Since scrapie has now been studied by competent

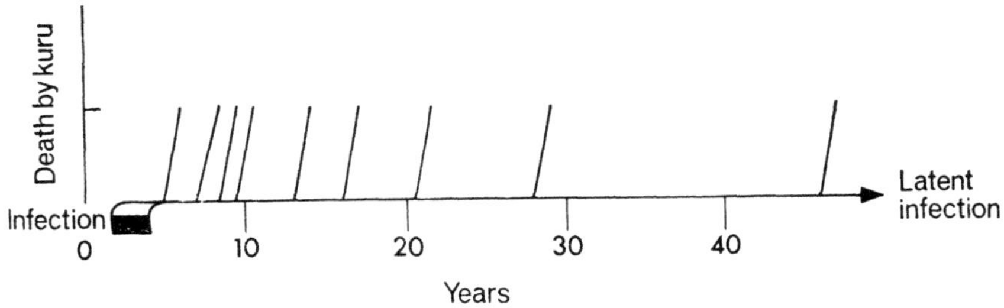

FIG. 15. Onset of kuru in relation to infection. To illustrate the need for a trigger to initiate symptomatic kuru: constructed from records of male deaths on the assumption that infection was in early childhood.

workers for several years, one must give considerable weight to their failure to demonstrate a conventional virus.

Kuru has some manifest resemblances to scrapie, but one cannot expect detailed studies of a virus whose existence can only be demonstrated by its power to induce disease in chimpanzees with an incubation period of a year or more. There is a hint that, as in scrapie, no neutralizing antibodies are present in the blood of infected subjects. Obviously there is much still to be learnt about the nature of the transmissible agent; as yet neither scrapie nor kuru can legitimately be called a virus disease.

In a recent discussion of kuru I have laid much weight on the fact that an 'infected' (predisposed) individual may be perfectly healthy for twenty years or more from her last episode of cannibalism and then, once the initial symptoms appear, the fatal course of the disease is completed within a year. What interrupts the 'persistent tolerated infection' by pulling a trigger, as it were, which sets the lethal cerebellar process into action? The only analogies available come from malignant disease and auto-immune disease, viz. that the condition is due to the appearance of a potentially pathogenic mutant cell and its proliferation. My own wholly speculative answer is to assume, first, that there is something which operationally one must call a virus, which can enter the body, proliferate, and persist without causing symptoms. Second, that for some reason the Purkinje cells of the cerebellum are vulnerable to auto-immune attack and that, once a casual T-immunocyte of appropriate specificity damages a Purkinje cell in a person harbouring the kuru virus, the trigger has been pulled. The damaged cell is vulnerable to the kuru virus, more 'cerebellar antigen' is liberated, and the appropriate T-immunocytes are stimulated to multiply. In some such fashion an autocatalytic lethal process associated with virus in the affected area can be visualized.

This interpretation is far from satisfactory. For one thing, there is no lymphocytic infiltration. The abundant cells are astrocytes and we know nothing about *their* possible immunological functions. We must confess in fact that the attempt to think of kuru as a persistent tolerated virus infection, triggered into lethal cerebellar degeneration by the development of auto-immune disease directed against a cerebellar antigen, has two inescapable weaknesses. The 'virus' has none of the accepted character of a virus and the postulated auto-immune process has none of the accepted histological concomitants.

I do not wholly rule out the possibility that some unforeseen development may make the analogy more relevant than it seems at present. It may become significant that an immunological deficiency disease, ataxia-telangiectasia, shows its main sympton from cerebellar degeneration. In the rare cases of cerebellar degeneration associated with gastric carcinoma or other cancers, the most likely hypothesis is the heterotopic production of cerebellar antigen by the tumour and auto-immune attack on the target organ.

Obviously a great deal more must be learnt about the nature of the transmissible agent in scrapie and kuru and about the possibilities of localized auto-immune attack in the central nervous system before the pathogenesis of this group of diseases is elucidated. All that can be said is that, particularly in kuru, the age incidence demands a stochastic interpretation that points more toward the emergence of a mutant clone of somatic cells than in any other direction.

CHAPTER 7

Auto-immune responses in normal animals

Basically there are two ways by which auto-immune disease can be simulated in genetically normal experimental animals. The animals can be immunized or sensitized by injection of cells or tissue extracts of other individuals of the same or a not too distantly related species. If immunization is done with the antigen emulsified in Freund's complete adjuvant and repeated injections given, auto-antibodies can be fairly regularly produced and not infrequently lymphocytic infiltration of the target organ occurs.

The second approach is rather clearly related to the forbidden clone concept. This is to inject a relatively large number of active lymphocytes from one animal, *A*, into another, *B*, which for one reason or another cannot mount an immune response against the *A* cells. In general, any animal will have in its circulation a significant proportion of lymphocytes which will react against tissue antigens of any unrelated animal of the same species. When the *A* cells are injected into *B*, some of them will 'recognize' antigenic determinants not present in *A* and be subject to the same probabilities of stimulation and reaction as a clone of auto-immunocytes produced by *B*. As a result, a characteristic disease picture can develop, commonly referred to as graft versus host reaction and sometimes as runt disease or homologous disease.

The commonest procedure is to inject parental cells into an F_1 animal. *AA* cells injected into an *AB* animal can react against the foreign antigen *B*, but *AB* cells accept *A* antigen as normal and hence do not react against the grafted cells.

Both approaches can throw light on some aspects of spontaneously occurring auto-immune disease.

Freund's complete adjuvant (*FCA*)

The standard statement that a vertebrate will not produce antibody or other immune response against its own substance has been subject to qualification ever since Uhlenhuth, in 1903, showed that lens protein from the same species could produce precipitins in rabbits. The introduction of FCA greatly increased the possibilities and, as Paterson has remarked, modern work on experimental auto-immunity is essentially a creation of Freund's adjuvant. The classical instance is the production of auto-immune encephalomyelitis in rats and other experimental animals by inoculation of extracts of central nervous system material with FCA. Extensive research on the nature of the antigen led first to the isolation of an encephalitogenic protein and then to the recognition that a peptide segment of the protein containing only sixteen amino acids could be effective. Active material can be obtained from any type of mammalian brain, but only under exceptional conditions does it show any effect if it is injected without adjuvant.

The role of FCA is clearly crucial. This is a water-in-oil emulsion containing killed acid-fast bacteria, usually tubercle bacilli, in which the antigen is emulsified by the use of a suitable surface-active emulsifier. Subcutaneous injection of this complex mixture results in the appearance of a substantial granulomatous swelling made up of a wide variety of inflammatory cells, including lymphocytes and plasma cells. Fibrous tissue develops and much of the inoculum is held in the lesion for a long period. Paraffin microglobules and antigen will, however, always be found in the draining lymph nodes as well.

The method is almost universally used by any investigator who desires to obtain high titre antibody with regularity as well as in all attempts to produce auto-antibodies or localized auto-immune disease in experimental animals. The function of the adjuvant is undoubtedly complex, involving not only the local granuloma but also the draining lymph nodes. Factors involved almost certainly include the slow release of antigen to the general circulation. Some antigen may reach the blood in soluble form, but it is equally likely that portion will be carried by cells leaving the granuloma by lymph channels and ending up in draining lymph nodes or reaching the spleen and other lymphoid tissues via the blood. On previous occasions I have speculated on the possibility that stem cells from the bone marrow might find in the granuloma a suitable environment for differentiation to T-immunocytes but not such a suitable one for any censorship function, so allowing occasional self-reactive or unduly avid immunocytes to pass to the circulation. Any evidence for this is indirect.

Auto-antibodies: the hapten-carrier hypothesis

Antibody is so much more readily assayed and investigated than specifically reactive cells that most work on experimental auto-immunity has been concerned with the production of auto-antibodies. There are two basic findings; *first*, that unless FCA is used there is at most only a trivial immune response to the injection of tissue extracts from the same species or even from another species of mammal; *second*, while tissues from an animal of the same strain and species give extracts which in general produce no antibody, similar extracts of the same tissues from another species are immunogenic. The antibody produced is tissue-specific and will react with extracts of tissue from both the donor of the immunogen and the animal making the antibody. It is therefore legitimate to speak of such an antibody as auto-antibody, although it cannot be produced in response to the animal's own tissue extract.

The most commonly accepted interpretation of this finding at the present time is that specific tissue antigens can be regarded as hapten-carrier composites, the hapten (H) being tissue-specific and rarely reaching the circulation; the carrier (C) is species- or strain-specific and possibly common to a number of combinations. There is full tolerance to C in the sense that no T- or B-immunocytes actively reactive with C are in circulation. For reasons which may be concerned either with the inaccessibility of H or because of its non-repetitive chemical character, H is neither immunogenic nor capable of producing tolerance, i.e. any B-immunocytes whose receptors can potentially react with H are neither stimulated nor destroyed. When, however, the corresponding tissue antigen C′–H from another species is injected with FCA, the current interpretation is that C′, being different from C, will find and stimulate T-immunocytes that can react with it. This reaction of C′–H with an anti-C′ immunocyte is essential if H is to make effective contact with an antibody-producing B-immunocyte and stimulate it to form a plasma cell clone. I am not satisfied that any adequate explanation of how this is effected has been given. I have tended to take the simplest interpretation that when C′–H antigen is constantly present in an environment through which immunocytes of all kinds are passing, an anti-H B-immunocyte will sooner or later find itself in the immediate vicinity of an anti-C′ T-immunocyte reacting with several units of C′–H. This will subject the B-immunocyte to non-specific stimulation by pharmacologically active agents arising from the C′-cell interaction and to specific stimulation by the H-antigenic determinant. By hypothesis this stimulates the B-cell to initiate an actively proliferating plasma cell clone. A tissue-specific antibody (anti-H) is in the making which will necessarily also react with H–C and be recognizable as an auto-antibody.

Intuitively I feel this is a vastly over-simplified account, but the mechanism described is based on some well-studied H–C models and may well represent a major component of what actually takes place or at least is the most useful mental picture to use in discussing clinical or experimental findings. In the preceding chapter (p. 92) the Wassermann reaction has been explained according to the same convention. Although for obvious reasons it is a less-popular interpretation, my own picture of the situation is that the H–C element is only a small part of the complexity of all experimental and clinical situations in this field. All tolerance is partial. Every immunoglobulin combining site, whether on immuno-receptor or on free antibody, can react with varying affinity to a wide range of antigenic determinants. An animal tolerant to antigenic determinant *A* can, in principle, only be legitimately compared with a normal animal by presenting two histograms showing the number or proportions of T and B immuno-receptors with each of, say, eight degrees of affinity for *A* (see Fig. 11). Whether or not the occasional immunocyte with moderate reactivity in the tolerant animal will be stimulated to proliferate by contact with antigen will depend on many factors, all of them representing probabilities rather than determinative influences.

An important point to be emphasized is that if (because of its inaccessibility or for any other reason) the tissue-specific determinant H is not capable of establishing tolerance, then any population of specific anti-H immunocytes will equally be incapable of reacting damagingly with the form in which the antigenic determinant is present in the body. An indication that true tolerance for tissue-specific antigens is possible in some organs can be seen in the work of Rose *et al.* with rabbit pancreas extracts. They immunized rabbits and examined for precipitins in the serum. When antibodies were produced they were never capable of reacting with extracts subsequently made from the injected animal's own pancreas. The overall results obtained conformed to the assumption that each rabbit pancreas carried either two or three of four antigens, A, B, C, D, and could produce only antibody against the one or two missing antigens.

This carrier-hapten interpretation fits well enough with most of the experimental findings, but it is not immediately applicable to auto-immune disease. An elderly woman with Hashimoto's disease of the thyroid has not been injected with rabbit thyroid in FCA. The full discussion of tissue-specific auto-immune disease must be left for a later section, but it is appropriate to suggest here that on the C–H convention for the structure of tissue antigens the essential requirement for auto-immune activity is inadequate tolerance for C.

In a good proportion of cases Hashimoto's disease may be preceded by toxic goitre with release of potential thyroid antigens, perhaps in the C–H form. It seems reasonable that all anti-C immunocytes should be subject to tolerance because of the high probability that the C components of all tissue antigens will have antigenic determinants found also in some accessible antigens. Any emergence of an anti-C immunocyte in a mutant form insusceptible to the tolerigenic action of the corresponding antigenic determinant will therefore provide an opportunity to allow (as in the experimental situation) the production of anti-H as a recognizable auto-antibody against a thyroid component. Again there is no intrinsic reason why antibody should have any damaging effect on the thyroid, and it is reasonable that we should find, as we do, that many more persons have thyroid auto-antibodies than show any sign of thyroid disease.

Experimental auto-immune encephalomyelitis

At this point we must return to auto-immune encephalomyelitis (AE) in experimental animals. Paterson and others have been unwilling to exclude the possibility that antibody may play a part, either positive or negative, in the production of the lesions in the central nervous system (CNS). It may be premature to ascribe AE wholly to the action of pathogenic T-immunocytes and to interpret the CNS lesions as essentially delayed hypersensitivity reactions to an antigenic determinant placed there by nature instead of being injected by the investigator. The evidence suggests strongly, without being decisive, that antibody of the same specificity as the aggressive immunocytes is produced to a variable extent by the injection of active material. It is particularly interesting that when Paterson's two strains of rat, Wistar and Lewis, were tested, Wistar showed mild encephalomyelitis and active production of antibody, while Lewis suffered severely, often lethally, from the T-immune attack and produced no antibody detectable by the complement fixation test being used.

Set experiments showed that the protective effect of antibody suggested by these findings could be directly demonstrated by passive administration of antiserum. The effect of antibody in specifically diminishing an immune response to the corresponding antigen is well known and has been referred to earlier. The simplest interpretation is that if a target is exposed to the entry of specifically reactive T-immunocytes it is even more exposed to any antibody that may be circulating. If the antibody can combine with surface antigenic determinants without damaging the target cell, it will automatically remove the points of contact that allow a T-immunocyte to damage the cell. The other possibility of an inhibitory effect depends on the capacity of antibody to mop up antigen, rendering it unavailable as an immunogenic stimulus (Fig. 16).

The pathogenesis of the brain or spinal cord lesion is not fully established, but there is no doubt that the lesion is basically an infiltration of mononuclear cells, lymphocytes, and monocytes from the circulation into the CNS substance. The possible mechanism by which this occurs in AE has already been discussed in relation to pharmacological aspects of immune responses in Chapter 5. There the suggestion was made that the cells of capillaries passing through an organ carry some organ-specific material which can serve as potential antigen. Any such antigenic determinants presenting on the surface of the capillary lumen would make the lining specifically sticky for sensitized immunocytes. Very little modification would be necessary if the primary event were fixation of high-affinity antibody, irritation by antigen-antibody-complement with permeability changes and non-specific stickiness, allowing a secondary involvement of both sensitized and non-specific cells. Some theoretical difficulties will also arise if what are often spoken of as tissue-specific inaccessible antigens not subject to tolerance are in fact always present in adjacent capillary endothelium and almost certainly moving still

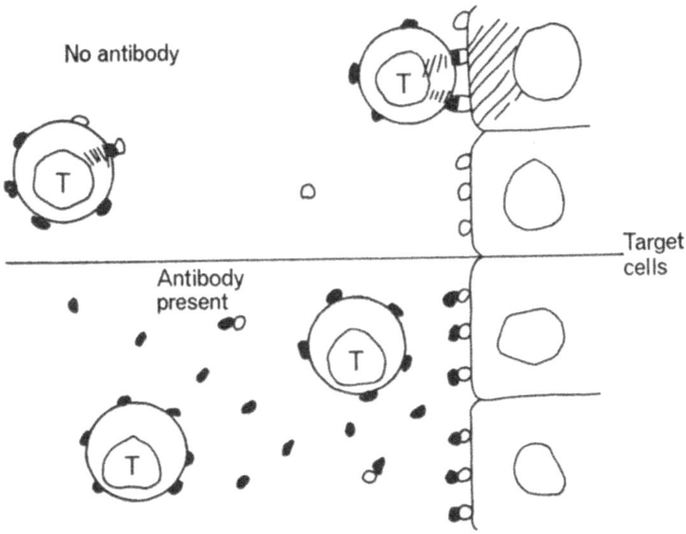

FIG. 16. Antibody as protection against T-cell action. T-immunocytes and antibody active against a target tissue are shown. If the target cell antigen is blocked by antibody neither stimulation of T-cells to proliferation nor their damaging action on the target cell is possible.
• = Antibody or immunocyte receptor. o = Target for antigen. Shading = damage to target cell or proliferative stimulus to T-cell.

further into other regions of the body. The C–H formulation in which tolerance to H is of no importance may well cover most of the difficulties, but it must be borne in mind that the nature of C and H in tissue extract antigens are still wholly undefined.

Experimental models of local auto-immune disease

The first example of a satisfactory imitation of local auto-immune disease in an experimental animal was Witebsky's production of thyroiditis in the rabbit. It was shown that even a rabbit's own thyroid tissue, obtained by surgical removal of half the gland, could be used as antigen with FCA to produce dense, small cell infiltration in the remaining thyroid tissue. In this instance it is not necessary to use tissue from a different species to obtain the auto-immune response. Such injections also produced anti-thyroid antibodies consistently, even in the minority of animals which failed to show infiltration of the thyroid with lymphocytes and plasma cells. At the time of their report, Witebsky's group was rather concerned to ascribe pathogenicity to the antibody produced, but the current approach would be to see the discrepancy as indicating that both T and B systems are usually concerned. On occasion, either for genetic reasons or by simple random failure of reactive immunocytes to appear, there is a sharp discrepancy of response between the two systems.

When experimentally injected animals are tested both for the development of delayed hypersensitivity (by skin test) and for circulating antibodies, several investigators have found a closer correlation of thyroiditis and cellular infiltration with delayed hypersensitivity to thyroglobulin than to antibody production.

Experimental auto-immune damage to the adrenal can also be produced by injection of a homogenate of one adrenal into the same individual guinea-pig. In these experiments, glands from other individuals seemed to be rather less active (Steiner, 1960). In rabbits, however, the usual rule held that only adrenals from other species produced the characteristic lesions.

Perhaps it is salutary to remember that if a rabbit is repeatedly injected with almost any potential antigen plus FCA it will eventually become sick, with a variety of auto-antibodies in the circulation and cellular infiltrates in many organs. Sometimes the animal reaches a condition reminiscent of systemic lupus in man. In all probability, intense enough artificial stimulation will allow immune responses to a wide variety of potential antigens which would be wholly ineffective if made available in physiological amounts. It also seems implicit from the results that there is no single process by which it is ensured that self components are non-immunogenic. It is probably always a fail-safe situation with co-operation between different mechanisms. One of the functions of some T-immunocytes, for instance, may be to recognize and destroy potentially pathological mutant immunocytes as part of the immunological surveillance function of the body. These fail-safe concepts will be elaborated in Chapter 12.

Graft-versus-host reaction as a model of auto-immune disease

In early experiments on inducing tolerance to skin grafts in mice the standard technique was to inject new-born mice of strain *A* with cells from spleen of a *B*-strain mouse. If the experiment went according to plan, by the time *A* was six weeks old it would accept a graft of *B* skin. With many combinations, however, the recipient of the foreign cells showed marked failure of growth, chronic diarrhoea, and other symptoms. This 'runt disease', or 'homologous disease', was especially liable to occur if spleen cells from an adult *B* mouse were used, less likely with adult bone marrow and least likely with the blood-cell-producing tissue of the liver in foetal or new-born mice.

It soon became evident that this graft-versus-host disease was an immune response by the donor cells against antigens in the recipient that were recognized as foreign. On the general hypothesis that we are adopting, if tolerance is to be induced by the classical method the immunocytes of both types must tolerate all alien antigens in the system. Any immunocytes of *B* (the donor) which are reactive with *A* antigens that are recognized as foreign must be eliminated and, conversely, any *A*-immunocytes reactive against an antigen carried on the *B*-cells of the inoculum must also be eliminated. Once this is accomplished, the two types can jointly occupy the lymphoid tissue to form a persisting chimera.

On this interpretation, it followed that by providing a one-sided advantage to the cell-donor a condition very like that postulated for auto-immune disease could be induced. The most convenient method, as indicated previously, was to inoculate into an F1 hybrid of two pure line strains (*AB*) cells from one parent, say *BB*. The genetic quality *B* is already present in the F1 recipient, so no immune response can be mounted. The foreign *BB* cells are therefore accepted as if they were genetically proper to the animal, just as 'auto-immune' cells arising spontaneously would be. The *BB* population, however, will contain a small proportion of immunocytes 'tuned' to react with the foreign antigens characteristic of the *A* component of the host. These cells will therefore have almost precisely the same immunological status as auto-immune cells and therefore are capable in principle of producing similar types of disease. With suitable strains and hybrids this can be shown to occur in rats, mice, and hamsters. Auto-immune haemolytic anaemia with positive Coombs test can often be produced and a variety of other antibodies. Chronic skin irritation and diarrhoea presumably represent the activity of *BB* cells on *A* components of the corresponding tissues.

Again in line with the standard interpretation, one must assume that when *BB* cells are injected it is only that small proportion which is reactive with an *A* antigen that proliferates and which, when an adequate population has been built up, is responsible for antibody production or for tissue damage. Since this point is a vital one for the understanding of auto-immune disease, it is worth while describing an experiment by Elkins which specifically establishes that this occurs.

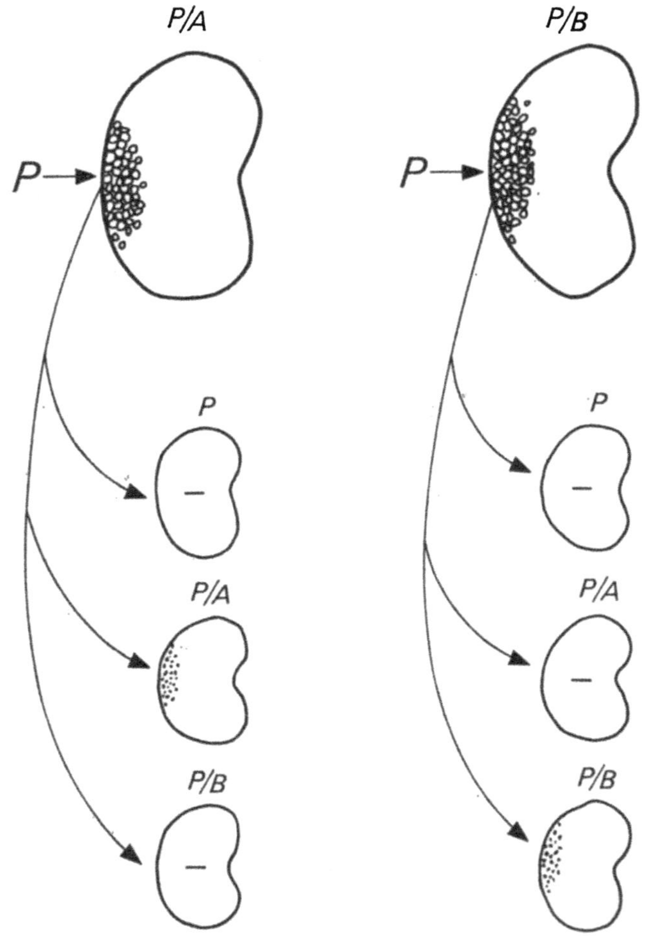

FIG. 17. Elkin's graft-versus-host experiment. Lymphocytes from rats of strain *P* were injected under the kidney capsule of F1 hybrids *P/A* and *P/B*. After some days the accumulated cells were tested similarly on rats of all three types with the results shown. See text for interpretation of the result.

He used a technique of injecting lymphocytes under the capsule of the rat's kidney, where most of them lodge at least for a few days. The occurrence of a graft-versus-host reaction is shown by proliferation of cells at the site to form a mass in which lymphocytes predominate. These lymphocytes can in their turn be tested for their power to produce a graft-versus-host reaction in other rats. Fig. 17 shows what happened when the lymphocytes accumulating after the primary inoculum of *P*-cells into F1 hybrids *P/A* and *P/B* were then tested in each of the three strains. Clearly, when *P*-cells were put under the capsule of a *P/A* kidney, it was only the immunocytes reactive against *A* which proliferated; any that reacted against *B* did not multiply and were diluted out or lost, so that, unlike the original *P* inoculum, this secondary inoculum had no effect on the *P/B* recipient. The same pattern of results was obtained with the other combination. Clearly, only immunocytes reactive with the antigen present in the host proliferated to produce the experimental analogue of a forbidden clone.

CHAPTER 8

The New Zealand mice

Ever since the concept of auto-immune disease was first advanced by Dameshek in 1937 investigators had felt the need for a better laboratory model than any of those that I have described in the previous chapter. In all of those, grossly unphysiological manipulations were needed to produce rather incomplete imitations of disease that arises, insidiously or acutely, but without any obvious 'cause' in man. What was needed was a strain of mice or guinea-pigs which with reasonable frequency spontaneously developed signs of auto-immune disease. In 1959 I heard through the late Sir Charles Hercus that a strain of mice had been developed in Dunedin (New Zealand) which regularly developed a positive Coombs test and signs of haemolytic anaemia. Since then the strain NZB and the F1 hybrid (NZB×NZW) have become the standard objects for experimental study of auto-immune disease throughout the world.

The NZ mouse strains were developed by Dr Marianne Bielschowsky in Dunedin. Bielschowsky and Goodall (1970) have recently summarized their origin. All are ultimately derived from mice of a mixed colour stock brought to New Zealand in 1930 from the Imperial Cancer Research Fund laboratories at Mill Hill. Three pairs of similarly coloured animals were picked with which to start inbred lines, while another white pair was similarly used by Hall at the Otago Medical School. The origins of the only three strains to be mentioned in this chapter were as follows.

From the agouti line some of the offspring had black coats and a brother–sister pair was used to initiate the *NZB* line. Haemolytic anaemia was observed from the eleventh generation onward. The original chocolate-coloured pair bred true for coat colour and became the *NZC* line. The white strain initiated by Mr W. H. Hall was developed as the pure line *NZW* and has been used in the breeding of F1 hybrids with NZB, which will be referred to as B/W mice.

Manifestations of auto-immune disease

The essential characteristic of the NZB strain is that some time after the age of 6 months the animals develop typical auto-immune haemolytic anaemia with positive direct Coombs (DC) test (see Fig. 19), moderate anaemia with a high reticulocyte count, and greatly enlarged spleen with much iron-containing debris (haemosiderosis). Many of the mice, particularly females, die with renal disease characterized by deposition of immunoglobulin, fibrinogen, and other blood proteins in relation to the glomerular basement membrane. In older mice splenic tumours are common, mostly of reticulum cell type.

All three aspects (haemolytic anaemia, renal disease, and late development of reticulum cell tumours) are regularly observed and are important for any interpretation of the condition. For the time being, however, it is convenient to put on one side the high incidence of tumours and the evidence in regard to the presence of low-grade possible oncogenic viruses.

NZB is the only laboratory strain of mice with a well-defined haemolytic anaemia of auto-immune type. Both sexes are involved and eventually almost 100 per cent give a positive antiglobulin test. In our hands there was a strikingly greater evidence of all the signs of haemolytic disease in males than in females. This difference has not been reported from other laboratories and it is not known whether the discrepancy is related to a genetic difference in our substrain or to some differences in husbandry. In other aspects of the haematological findings there is general agreement amongst the laboratories concerned. There is good reason to believe that the condition is a reasonable laboratory model of auto-immune haemolytic anaemia (warm type) in man.

The B/W hybrids are much shorter lived and in our experience the females died regularly from kidney disease before reaching the age of 400 days. Many of both sexes died without showing conversion to the Coombs-positive state, but results with survivors suggested that in the absence of kidney disease most mice would have shown a slow development of a positive Coombs test.

Apart from minor differences, all workers are agreed on these general attributes of the mice and it might have been expected that intensive work on both NZB and B/W mice since 1958 would by this time have solved the nature and pathogenesis of the disease. This is

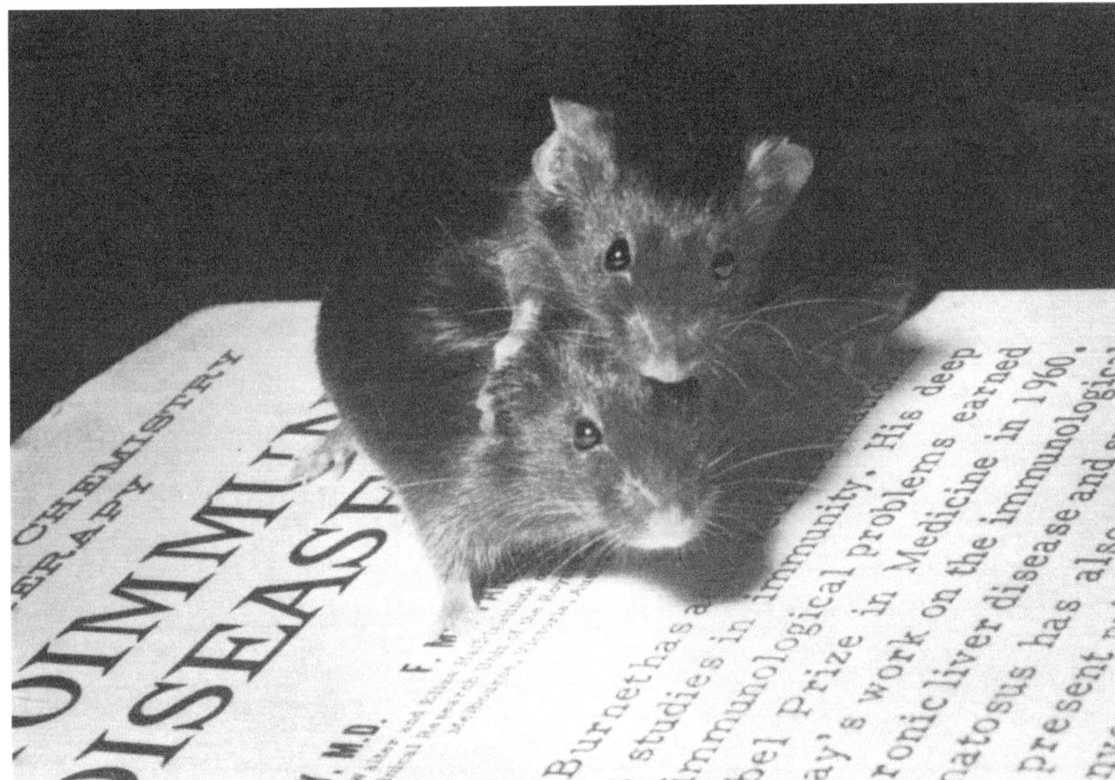

PLATE I. New Zealand Black (NZB) mice.

far from what has happened. At the present time there seem to be three general hypotheses still viable:

1. That the condition is due essentially to a vertically transmitted virus infection, the virus being closely related to murine oncogenic viruses of Type C.

2. That there is a genetically based functional abnormality by which these mice are hyper-responsive to antigens and less readily develop tolerance to any antigen. The nature of the abnormality and its relevance to the disease is still obscure.

3. That the mice are predisposed genetically to give rise to 'forbidden clones' highly reactive with red cell antigens.

If virus infection plays a part in the etiology of the condition, it must work by intruding into the genetic mechanism at either germinal or somatic level. It seems logical, therefore, to attempt to define the genetic situation before looking for any extrinsic agent that might have induced the genetic anomaly.

Genetic and somatic genetic factors

The regularity with which the DC test and other signs of the condition appear makes it certain that the disease is genetically determined. This, of course, does not necessarily exclude a hypothesis that it is due to a virus incorporated in some way in the host genome. Fairly extensive genetic studies have been made in several laboratories. Hybrids of NZB with standard strains such as C3H give much longer-lived mice, of which most of the females develop a positive DC test at a much later period of life. In the males the proportion is still smaller and most die without converting to Coombs positive. It may be of interest that when the age-specific incidence of conversion to a positive DC test is plotted log–log according to Burch's method, the straight lines expected for a population 100 per cent susceptible are obtained (Fig. 18).

Crosses with other NZ strains are more interesting. The chocolate-coloured mice of the NZC strain never show signs of auto-immunity, but when crossed with NZB the F1 offspring show the same early and regular development of the DC test. Warner has studied this and other NZB crosses in relation to other serological qualities and concludes that two unusual genes at distinct loci are relevant to the auto-immune condition. The first, present only in NZB, is dominant,

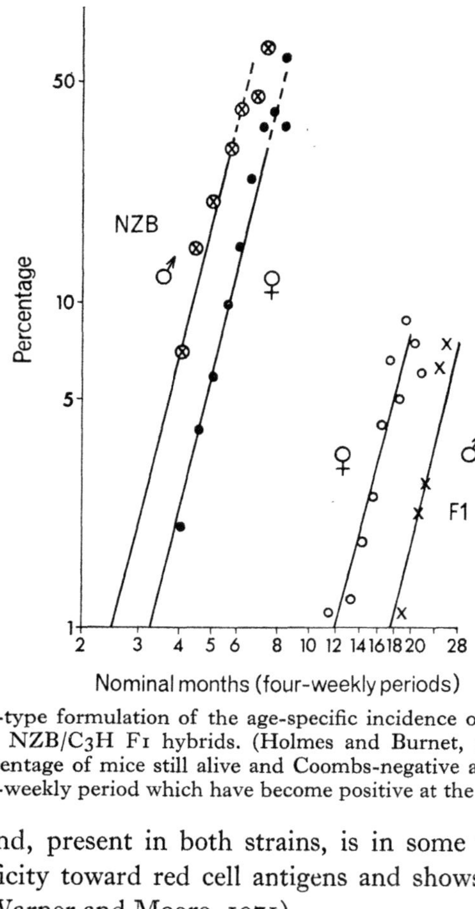

FIG. 18. A Burch-type formulation of the age-specific incidence of Coombs conversion in NZB and NZB/C3H F1 hybrids. (Holmes and Burnet, 1964.) The points represent the percentage of mice still alive and Coombs-negative at the beginning of each two-weekly period which have become positive at the end of it.

while the second, present in both strains, is in some way concerned with the specificity toward red cell antigens and shows a strong gene dosage effect (Warner and Moore, 1971).

Genetic factors are undoubtedly involved, but alone cannot provide any interpretation of the characteristic age incidence of Coombs conversion. On the working hypothesis we are using, this must depend on somatic mutation or some equivalent process. By far the most effective way of establishing the somatic genetic origin of an abnormal condition is to demonstrate that the cells concerned are of monoclonal origin in at least some examples of the condition. This has been successfully accomplished by Warner in work so far only published in the Hall Institute Annual Reports. In crosses between NZB and C57BL, the F1 generation showed late appearance of direct Coombs tests. Warner was specially interested in IgG2a immunoglobulins, which are allotypically distinct between these two strains. Of twenty sets of Coombs positive cells, only five were coated with this immunoglobulin. Three were specifically C57BL, two were NZB, none showed both. With NZC/NZB hybrids there were again very few with IgG2a coating the cells, but all were of only one parental type.

Obviously more extensive work to confirm these results is desirable, but there is no reason not to accept them as they stand as indicating that the auto-immune antibody responsible for the Coombs test is of monoclonal origin in at least a quarter of the mice. In other words, the population of cells producing the antibody responsible for the Coombs test was initiated by a single immunocyte. Admittedly the significant data come from the C57BL/NZB hybrids in which the Coombs test develops slowly and in which there could well be a better chance to detect a monoclonal situation. Nevertheless, if a condition is monoclonal in at least 5 out of 20 mice, it becomes highly probable that even the rapidly developing condition in NZB mice will involve only a few separate clones. As I have discussed earlier, monoclonal situations require a special approach to understanding their etiology.

Transfer to other mice

From the earliest stages of our work with NZB mice the main objective was to find a way of defining a set of cells as responsible for the immunopathological effects. Holmes *et al.* (1961) showed that transfer of spleen cells from Coombs positive animals to syngeneic young mice resulted in the rapid appearance of the Coombs positive state in the recipient. This sometimes remained until it merged into the usual development of a positive test as the animal aged, but sometimes the initial reaction faded and there was a negative interim period before the permanent establishment of the auto-immune condition. The results have been subsequently confirmed by Kay and Hook (1964) and by Holborrow *et al.* (1965). Cells from lymph nodes, bone marrow, and thymus were ineffective. This made it clear that the spleen at least contained many more of the effective cells than other possible sites.

In our experiments no positive results were obtained when the recipients were young mice of a different strain. This is not always the case. Allman *et al.* (1969) found that by transferring bone marrow from young adult NZB mice to new-born CBA recipients they could virtually replace the immune system with one of NZB quality. These chimeric recipents became Coombs positive after a few months. The results establish directly what any current hypothesis would probably assume, i.e. that the effective cells derive from stem cells in the bone marrow.

In an experiment which can be regarded as complementary to transfer, Lindsey and Woodruff (1967) heavily irradiated Coombs positive NZB mice and 'rescued' them with injections of bone marrow cells from young NZB or (NZB/CBA-T6) F1 hybrids. In the first group the mice became and remained Coombs negative for some months; in the second group, with the F1 cells, they remained persistently Coombs negative with at least 90 per cent bone marrow and lymphoid cells of donor karyotype.

Both the transfer and radiation experiments are in line with the preferred hypothesis that special clones of immunocytes derived from bone marrow stem cells are concerned. The application of more sophisticated modern methods was, however, clearly needed.

Plaque-forming cells

After a number of fruitless attempts by other workers, Wilson, Warner, and Holmes (1971) have been able to demonstrate auto-immune plaque-forming cells (PFC) against mouse red cells in old NZB mice. The great majority of the plaques obtained from the spleens of old Coombs positive NZB mice were IgM as were most of the Coombs antibodies. There were, however, some discrepancies between the immunoglobulin type of the plaques and of the Coombs antibody. It is probably significant that high counts of PFC were confined to the spleen and increased in relation to the age of the mouse and size of the spleen. Roughly a 10-fold increase in spleen size was associated with 120-fold increase in plaque-forming cells. In young mice still Coombs negative, small numbers of PFC were regularly present in the spleen. It is in line with this that Warner has been able to show that immunization with allogeneic red cells given intravenously induced prematurely early positive Coombs tests in 58 per cent of young NZB mice.

Small numbers of PFC were present in the thymus of old mice (mostly IgG), but no more than in control mice of similar age, and none were found in bone marrow, mesenteric lymph nodes, or Peyer's patches.

These findings at the genetic and cytological levels are obviously of great significance, but it should be emphasized that so far they have not been confirmed in laboratories other than the Hall Institute. Discrepancies between the findings with different substrains of NZB have been common in the past and it seems urgent that some other stocks of NZB should be tested in similar ways.

Immunological vigour in NZB mice

The other important sets of findings wherein NZB mice differ functionally from others is in their higher capacity for response to certain antigens. Morton and Siegel (1969), for instance, find that, using the standard sheep red cell antigen and Jerne plaque-forming cell counts, the maximum count of PFC per spleen is from 2 to 20 times higher than other strains of mice. What may well be more significant is that, whereas with other strains there is an optimal size of immunizing dose, this does not hold with NZB mice. The larger the antigen dose (up to 10^9 cells), the higher is the plaque count. All these findings were on young adult NZB mice not yet Coombs positive. As in other strains, old mice are less immunologically active.

The same authors found that NZB mice are more radio-resistant when young than other strains with an LD50 (30 d) of 960 r at 4 weeks of age; but for old Coombs positive mice it is 540 r. Probably related to this is Warner and Moore's finding that in lethally irradiated NZB there were many more endogenous stem cells capable of producing clonal nodules (Till–McCulloch) in the spleen than in all other strains except NZC.

With most mouse strains, foreign gammaglobulin freed of aggregated particles produces immune paralysis (tolerance) against the usually immunogenic semi-denatured material. No tolerance can be produced in this way with adult NZB mice (Staples and Talal, 1969), and although tolerance can be induced in weanling mice, it is lost between 4 and 6 weeks. Another indication of the high immunological activity of the strain is the ease with which anti-nucleic acid antibodies are provoked by the synthetic poly-I-C polynucleotide. This is associated with an accelerated development of fatal glomerulonephritis (Steinberg *et al.*, 1969).

An important new character of NZB was recognized when Warner produced myelomatosis in NZB mice by intraperitoneal injection of mineral oil. The picture was basically similar to what is observed in BALB/c mice. BALB/c×NZB hybrids were equally susceptible but no other NZB hybrids gave positive results. It may be significant that Mason and Warner (1969/70) have noted a much higher tendency for secondary mutations to take place in the myeloma lines induced in NZB than in those from BALB/c mice. Both strains are of histocompatibility group $H2^d$, but many other mouse strains in the same group are not susceptible to myeloma induction. Warner has suggested that it may be relevant that NZB and BALB/c mice both fail to show Dresser's phenomenon of being immunologically paralysed by an injection of a foreign gammaglobulin freed from aggregates by prolonged centrifugation. Another finding due to Warner (personal communication) is that with the strains BALB/c and NZC, which never develop spontaneous Coombs reactions, injection of allogeneic red cells in Freund's complete adjuvant provoked a positive (DC) test in 40–100 per cent. This did not happen with syngeneic cells nor did allogeneic cells injected into other strains of mice provoke a Coombs reaction. This is generally in line with the phenomena of auto-antibody production, discussed in a previous section (p. 99).

Are viruses concerned?

The third approach is the now conventional one of ascribing any stochastically based pathological condition to a slow virus infection and very often finding a virus to fit. No one has claimed to have *proved* that the essential anomaly in NZB mice is the carriage and vertical transmission of an oncogenic murine virus, but this is clearly in the minds of several workers. There is no doubt that the NZB mice stocks used by Mellors and by East are associated with an oncogenic virus producing acute lymphomas. The Hall Institute substrain behaves differently, although, as will be described later, it does show a high tendency to develop tumours of lymphoma-reticulum cell sarcoma types. Russell *et al.* (1970) failed to find electron-microscopic evidence of virus particles and no one has been able to transmit the condition by filtrates of NZB spleens to any other strain of mice.

Over the years there have been extensive studies by Melbourne workers of the results of injecting suspensions of spleen cells into young mice of the NZB strain and other strains. The results of transfer to young Coombs negative NZB mice have been described already. Cells killed by freezing and thawing or by heat produced no effect in young syngeneic mice. Some of the early transfers of cells to young NZB mice by Holmes *et al.* (1961) occasionally resulted in the appearance of an acute lymphomatous condition with involvement of the thymus and transmissible to further syngeneic mice. This, however, was very unusual and was not subsequently observed. We were not specifically interested in the nature of the common reticulum cell tumour found in 20–30 per cent of old NZB mice autopsied after death or killed when moribund. What did interest us, although it has not been specifically studied, was the finding on several occasions of lymphomatous nodules in the spleen of mice which had been inoculated with splenic cells from a Coombs positive mouse. Transfer from one such tumorous spleen by intraperitoneal injection gave the same picture with macroscopically visible nodules wholly confined to the spleen. Retrospectively, this finding probably deserved more study than the few casual experiments which were made.

Pathogenesis of the auto-immune condition

There has been no general discussion of the pathogenesis of auto-immune haemolytic anaemia in NZB mice since the appearance of the work of Wilson *et al.*, so that it seems justifiable to present a short interpretation of the situation in the light of that work and the immunogenetic findings of Warner's group. Broadly, I would dismiss viruses as irrelevant and concentrate solely on genetic and somatic genetic processes. There can be no doubt that NZB mice possess some genes that are unique and we can accept Warner's interpretation of his NZB×NZC F1 studies as indicating that two of these genes involve separate loci.

A priori, everything suggests that the disease arises because an occasional cell undergoes somatic mutation which allows it to escape the normal controls which 'disallow' newly differentiated immunocytes potentially capable of damaging action on other body cells. In one hybrid which is considerably slower in becoming Coombs positive than pure line NZB mice the evidence is decisive that in five instances the Coombs antibody was monoclonal. In the typical NZB condition it is almost certainly not so since both IgM and IgG antibodies are involved. Another important point is the existence in normal mouse strains of a few plaque-forming cells of auto-immune type in older animals. Perhaps equally relevant is the result obtained by Norins and Holmes (1964) that mice of the random-bred Hall Institute strain show a steady increase with age in the proportion with antinuclear factor in their sera. This may be regarded as an auto-immune process, but there was no evidence that it was producing any signs of disease. It provides a good example of the principle that auto-immune disease can only develop when the clones of immunocytes concerned can break through a fail-safe system of multiple controls.

In the NZB mice the main factor which allows the escape and proliferation of the pathogenic clone(s) seems likely to be the weakness of one of the secondary controls. This is related to the well-established difficulty in rendering NZB mice specifically tolerant (or paralysed) by the administration of relatively large doses of antigen which are effective in other strains. It is of particular interest that Morton and Siegel (1969) found that the PFC response to sheep red cells in young NZB mice showed no evidence of an inhibitory effect by large doses of antigen. In brief, the most likely interpretation of the genetic anomaly in NZB mice is a general resistance of immunocytes to the tolerigenic action of high doses of antigen. It would be in line with this to find that minor somatic mutation would more frequently give an additional resistance which would allow the emergence of a pathogenically active clone.

There is still need to seek some interpretation of the conspicuous concentration of auto-antibodies on the erythrocyte as target cell. The striking changes in the spleen and the high concentration of specific PFC cells there point strongly to some quality of the splenic environment being responsible.

In the normal spleen there is constant destruction of outdated red cells and, by implication, a high concentration of solubilized or partially solubilized red cell surface antigens. Such a concentration could be relied on to paralyse any occasional immunocyte which might lodge in the spleen with immune receptors reactive against autologous erythrocyte antigen. In the NZB spleen there is an accelerated destruction of the 'opsonized' Coombs positive cells and an even more massive liberation of antigenic material. Any mutant immunocytes resistant to inactivation by excess antigen and reactive with a common red cell antigen would be stimulated to proliferation under the circumstances.

We can reach the same conclusion by a slightly different route. The primary genetic anomaly in NZB mice is manifested in an abnormally high resistance of all immunocytes to destruction or inhibition by specific antigenic contact. This will imply that relatively minor mutations can raise that resistance still further in individual cells. For these to proliferate to pathogenic clones there will need to be at some accessible site relatively large amounts of the corresponding auto-antigen. Here the special position of the spleen as the main disposal site for effete red cells comes into the picture. Nowhere else in the body is there such an accumulation in various stages of breakdown of potential auto-antigen. Clearly there will be a premium for selective proliferation of cells with auto-immune potentiality which can react with a common red cell antigen.

CHAPTER 9

Diseases primarily involving blood cells

AUTO-IMMUNE HAEMOLYTIC ANAEMIA

The general concept of auto-immune disease began to take form in 1938 with Dameshek's and Schwartz's demonstration of haemolysin in some patients with acute haemolytic anaemia. Real advances only came, however, when the technique that Coombs, Mourant, and Race had developed to detect incomplete Rh antibodies (the direct Coombs test) was applied to patients with various types of haemolytic anaemia.

Clinically and serologically, the main feature of auto-immune haemolytic anaemia (AHA) is its heterogeneity. The disease can be defined as a persisting anaemia, with no toxic or other cause apparent, associated with a direct Coombs test and usually a high level of reticulocytes. The direct Coombs test is carried out by testing washed red cells from the patient with dilutions of anti-human gammaglobulin produced by rabbit immunization. Positive agglutination represents a positive direct Coombs test (DC+). Such a result indicates that the patient's red cells are coated with an antibody-like protein of relatively low affinity for the corresponding antigenic determinant on the red cell surface. Although firmly enough bound to the coated cell, the Coombs antibody cannot form bridges between two cells and so build up the aggregates of cells which are seen in agglutination reactions.

Serum from a rabbit immunized with pooled globulins from human serum will contain sufficient high affinity antibody molecules reacting with antigenic determinants on immunoglobulins (and some other human blood proteins) to link the coated cells together. By using specially prepared antisera specific for individual antigens associated with human immunoglobulins κ, λ, μ, and γ, it is possible to define the types of immunoglobulin involved in rendering the red cells Coombs positive or to demonstrate that the protein involved is not an immunoglobulin.

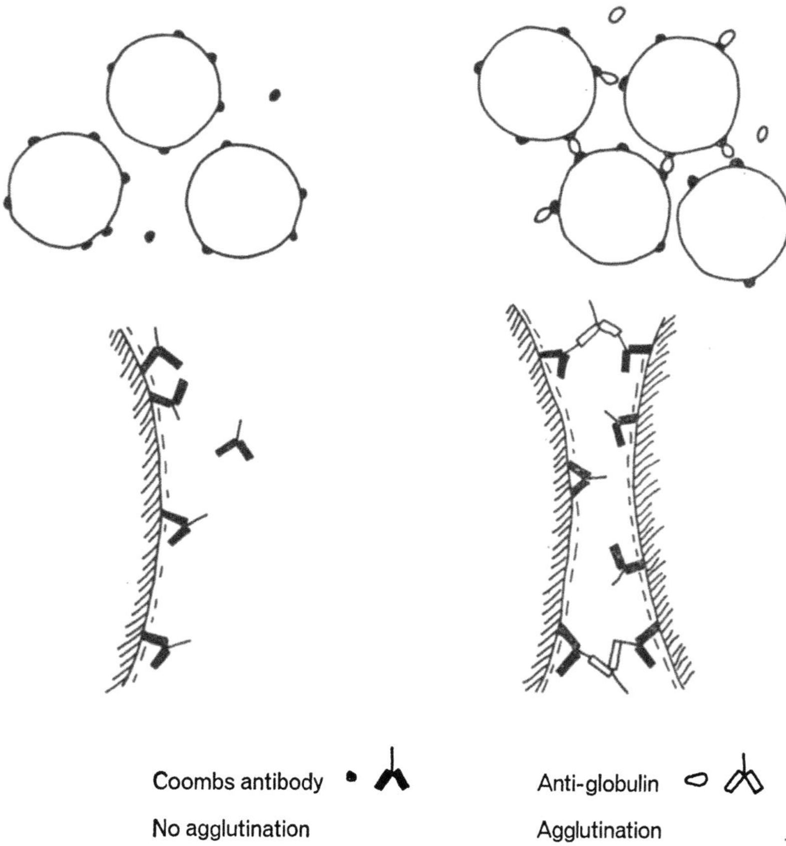

FIG. 19. Interpretation of the Coombs (anti-globulin) test. The auto-antibody is of relatively low affinity and partially obstructed by the layer of glycoprotein on the red cell surface. It does not normally cause agglutination but the immunoglobulin molecules are firmly attached to the red cell surface. When a rabbit antiserum against human immunoglobulin is added to the system, the anti-globulin molecules act as bridges which can hold red cells in contact and so cause agglutination. Antibody molecules are shown according to the current convention for IgG in the 'high power' diagram; the combining sites of the anti-globulin molecules unite with the Fc portion of the auto-antibody molecules. A discontinuous layer of loosely attached protein is also indicated.

From the laboratory angle, cases of auto-immune haemolytic anaemia are primarily divided into those with 'warm type' antibodies and those with 'cold type'. Some 90 per cent of cases of idiopathic cases of haemolytic anaemia can be clearly differentiated into one or other type, but virtually every serum has some unique immunological qualities and a small proportion show anomalous temperature reactions.

Warm type AHA

The commoner form, the so-called warm type, shows no spontaneous agglutination or haemolysis in drawn blood. The cold type shows agglutination as the blood cools and the washed cells are spontaneously agglutinated below some temperature varying with the patient but generally around 28 – 32 °C. When tested at 37 °C the cells give a DC+ of 'non-gammaglobulin' type, presumably associated with the adsorption of complement components.

Most of the discussion will be concerned with the warm type of auto-immune haemolytic anaemia. The disease can occur at any age including infancy. In very young children it can be very acute and is fatal in about a third of the cases. In some, recovery is spontaneous and rapid. At all ages there is great variability in the course of the disease, but in general the mortality is high. In a carefully studied and treated series Dacie had a mortality of 46 per cent.

Secondary AHA is most commonly seen as a sequel to a chronic proliferative disease of the lymphoid system, chronic lymphocytic leukaemia, reticulosarcoma, or lymphoma. The only other common secondary type is associated with systemic lupus erythematosus.

Immunological features

The first point to be emphasized is that there is no intrinsic abnormality in the blood cells of the patient. Labelled blood, transfused from a normal compatible donor, is destroyed at the same rate as the patient's own. The accelerated blood cell destruction takes place in the spleen, but it is not clearly known what part the antibody coating plays or whether active cell-mediated destruction in the spleen is significant. Most of the discussion of pathogenesis in AHA will be left for Chapter 13. Here we will be mainly concerned with the types of antibody demonstrable in the blood or adsorbed to the circulating cells.

It is highly characteristic of AHA that each patient's serum seems to have its own individual quality. This probably holds just as strongly for all auto-immune diseases, but the degree to which serological work with human red cells can be elaborated and refined allows it to be specially evident with AHA. The most striking finding is that the red cell antigenic determinants involved are never the well-known ones concerned in iso-agglutinin reactions between different individuals. About a third of the antibodies can be shown to be specific for one of the Rh antigens, most often anti-e or anti-c. Most react with all unselected human red cells, but when tested with cells from the very rare genotypes -D-/-D- or ---/--- many antibodies fail to react. Even with the completely deleted cells (from a single Australian aborigine) about 40 per cent of active AHA sera will react. Another interesting feature is that sera from AHA cases will often recognize 'private' antigens, i.e. an antigen, recognized by some immune serum, which is present only in one individual or a group of close relatives.

It is rare to see auto-agglutination of the patient's own red cells at 37 °C or haemolysis. However, in a series of more then 80 cases Dacie found that sera from 4 patients agglutinated normal red cells at 37 °C and 2 of these also produced haemolysis. Red cells treated with trypsin or papain are agglutinated by many more sera (55 out of 84) than are normal human red cells. In all probability this results from the antigenic determinants on the red cell surface becoming more accessible to the combining site of antibody as a consequence of the removal of superficial protein. Haemolysis of trypsinized red cells was observed with 15 out of 84 sera from AHA patients.

In all probability these results point to a wide range of affinity of the antibody combining sites for the red cell antigenic determinants. It is perhaps worth underlining here that as in so many immunological situations there is no predetermined correspondence between AD on red cell and combining site on antibody or immune receptor; effects are produced only when the two patterns 'happen to fit'. A sterically complementary fit can be of varying degrees of affinity or 'goodness of fit' and the observable consequences cover a corresponding spectrum of intensity.

From the point of view of a theoretical understanding of the auto-immune process, a particularly important feature is the evidence pointing to monoclonal origin of antibody in AHA. Leddy and Bakemeier (1965) showed that of 21 samples of antibody eluted from DC+ cells from as many patients with warm type AHA, 11 contained only K light chains, 4 contained L, 2 were unequivocally mixed K and L, while the other 4 were also probably mixed. There is no other reasonable interpretation of this finding than a monoclonal origin in about 50 per cent of cases.

Cold type AHA

The cold type disease is much rarer than warm type AHA and is largely confined to the older age-groups. It is usually chronic and associated with only minor degrees of anaemia, sometimes with characteristically lower haemoglobin values in winter. A proportion of patients show signs of Raynaud's disease (painful fingers, ears, etc., associated with local circulatory weakness) and haemoglobinuria in very cold weather. Both symptoms are believed to be due to plugging of capillaries by agglutinated red cell aggregates and haemolysis in regions with a sharply lowered tissue temperature.

The low-grade antibody which is present in these cases, often in very large amount, is always of low affinity in the sense that it never causes agglutination of the patient's cells at 37 °C. It is directed against a curious antigenic determinant present on 99·9 per cent of red cells obtained from human adults. Foetal red cells obtained from the umbilical cord at the time of birth, however, are almost unsusceptible to agglutination by such sera. The conventional statement is that all infants are born with red cells carrying the antigen (or AD) *i*, but within a month or two all cells change, so that *i* becomes, or is replaced by, *I* antigen. In less than 0·1 per cent of people the change of *i* to *I* fails to occur and all cells remain *i* and therefore virtually unagglutinated by sera from these patients with cold type AHA.

A further point of interest is that all the cold agglutinins are immunoglobulins with K type light chains. Evidence that the disease is of monoclonal origin can still be drawn from the fact that only one subgroup, most often *K*III but sometimes *K*I or *K*II, is present.

At room temperature (±20 °C) many sera cause haemolysis as well as agglutination of *I* cells from any individual. As the temperature is raised, the strength of agglutination weakens, and by the time 37 °C is reached nearly all show aggregates disappearing to leave a smooth suspension of evenly dispersed red cells. Occasionally a serum will still agglutinate some human *I* red cells at 37 °C but never those from the same patient.

A distinct though possibly related haemolytic disease has been known since the middle of the nineteenth century as paroxysmal cold haemoglobinuria; it was usually seen as a rare manifestation of congenital syphilis in children. In 1904 Donath and Landsteiner showed that there was an amboceptor (antibody) in the blood which became attached to the patient's (or any other human) red cells at temperatures below 18 °C. Ever since, this has been known as the Donath–Landsteiner, or D–L, antibody. When the coated cells were then warmed in the presence of complement, they were rapidly dissolved. The clinical picture of episodes of passing urine deeply coloured with haemoglobin after exposure to cold is accounted for by union of auto-antibody and red cells when blood is passing through the vessels of chilled hands or feet and lysed as it is rewarmed on return to the heart. As in all such conditions, there are wide clinical and serological variations from case to case and some have features that bring them close to the cold haemagglutinin type of haemolytic anaemia. Serologically, there is a sharp difference, since the D–L antibody reacts with all human cells and is not limited, as cold haemagglutinin is, to cells carrying antigen *I*.

For anyone interested in a forbidden clone theory of auto-immune disease, the etiology of the condition is of particular interest. There can be no doubt about the frequent association with congenital syphilis, but in Dacie's view there are undoubtedly cases in non-syphilitics. Some are said to have followed measles, infectious mononucleosis, or other minor infection. Probably all that it is justifiable to claim is that the condition is a rare sequel even of congenital syphilis and therefore could well represent the emergence of a mutant immunocyte clone. In one case of Dacie's a young man with no evidence of syphilis showed a typical isolated episode of haemoglobinuria and then remained free of any symptoms for eight years, although his D–L antibody remained demonstrable throughout. This must mean that the antibody-producing cells derived their anomalous quality from a genetic change, possibly of germinal origin but much more likely resulting from somatic mutation. There is no real basis for speculating how congenital treponemal infection could induce a particular type of somatic mutation, but equally there is no reason why any intracellular, non-cytotoxic infection by virus, treponema, or any other micro-organism should not increase the likelihood of somatic mutation. I have recently discussed this approach in another context (Burnet, 1971).

THROMBOCYTOPENIC PURPURA

Without attempting to discuss the very complex mechanism concerned with blood coagulation and the control of minor bleeding, it can be said that if the circulating platelets (thrombocytes) fall below 60,000 per mm^3 (normal $\pm$300,000) the individual is liable to show small patches of haemorrhage into the skin. Similar haemorrhages may occur in other organs, sometimes with the production of symptoms. This is the condition known clinically as thrombocytopenic purpura. This clinical picture has already been described as a result of the administration of quinidine and some other drugs.

The same picture is seen without any obvious inciting cause as idiopathic thrombocytopenic purpura (ITP), a disease seen mainly in children and young women, which is widely considered to be of auto-immune character. The important clinico-pathological features of the disease are, first, the evidence that a blood serum factor, presumably an auto-antibody, is responsible for platelet destruction, and, second, that splenectomy frequently allows an increase in platelets and sometimes appears to provide a definitive cure.

It has proved very difficult to give a clear demonstration of antibodies causing platelet agglutination oı lysis, though there are many claims that factors capable of these actions are present in serum from ITP patients. The most cogent evidence comes from placental transmission of the disease from mother to child. There is a tendency for symptoms to be accentuated in pregnancy and in 35–68 per cent of instances the infant shows haemorrhages during the first weeks of life. The congenital disease can be fatal as a result of intracranial bleeding. Since IgG antibody readily crosses the placenta, while cells from the mother do not, and since the haemorrhages cease to occur in the infant after 4–12 weeks this almost establishes IgG auto-antibody as a major factor in the pathogenesis of the disease. Pointing in the same direction is the fact that normal platelets, administered intravenously to a patient, rapidly disappear from the circulation. The most direct demonstration of antibody was by the use of ITP plasma given intravenously to normal volunteers, with a rapid fall in the level of circulating platelets (Shulman *et al.*, 1965).

Platelets, like red cells, appear to be removed from circulation at the end of their useful life by being taken up in the spleen. Everything suggests that in ITP the platelets, sensitized by auto-antibody, have a greatly shortened life in the circulation before being removed by the spleen. Again, the most direct experiments are those of Shulman *et al.*, who administered the same ITP plasma to two volunteers who had been splenectomized and a normal individual. There was no fall in platelet count in the absence of a spleen in contrast to the precipitate fall in the normal person. Splenectomy is a standard form of treatment in any persisting case of ITP and in many instances the platelet count rises and haemorrhages disappear. In some patients the operation is ineffective and the platelet count may remain low. Such failures were shown in Shulman's experiments to be associated with a higher degree of sensitization by antibody of higher affinity, so allowing the platelets to be actively removed by the liver even in splenectomized individuals.

Basically, therefore, the situation in ITP is very similar to what is found in auto-immune haemolytic anaemia. The primary event is the emergence of immunocytes reactive with platelet antigenic determinants and relatively resistant to natural tolerance induction. Such immunocytes, certainly B- and probably also T-cells, lodge and proliferate predominantly in the spleen, where the platelet antigenic determinant will be in highest concentration. One could almost guarantee that if there were a way of titrating antibody-producing cells, the great majority would be found in the spleen, just as plaque-forming cells (PFC) are in NZB mice. In both human and murine AHAs the drain on red cell production in the bone marrow is shown by the number of reticulocytes in circulation. So in ITP, bone marrow smears show an excess of immature megakaryocytes.

Leukopenias and pancytopenias

Amongst iatrogenic diseases damage to bone marrow function occupies a very important place. It is mandatory, for instance, to carry out regular leucocyte counts in any patient treated with chloramphenicol or the cytotoxic drugs and advisable with many others. Sometimes the damaging effect can be reasonably ascribed to a directly toxic effect on the stem cells of the bone marrow. No drug which at the recommended dosage produces a high incidence (0·1 per cent or more) of bone marrow failure will be allowed to remain in the pharmacopoeia. With all those currently in use it is a rare complication, which means that in one way or another the unfortunate victim is anomalous. The functional lesion may be a genetically based anomaly in some metabolic function relevant to the action or the disposal of the drug or it may be the existence of anomalous clones of immunocytes with auto-immune capacity. Dausset, using his anti-gammaglobulin consumption test, concluded that a substantial proportion (23 per cent) of leukopenias ascribed to drugs were associated with auto-antibody directed against leucocytes. This was only slightly lower than the 29 per cent found in idiopathic leukopenia or aplastic anaemia. There is no evidence for or against the possibility that some or all of the cases without demonstrable antibody are due to the presence of auto-immune T-cells directed against stem cell components.

There is just not enough information available to justify speculation as to how chloramphenicol, for instance, produces fatal bone marrow failure in about 1:50,000 of those treated. If it were a common condition, a fairly complete answer could almost certainly be obtained by studies of the type used by Shulman to compare quinidine purpura with auto-immune ITP, but that is not possible with an excessively rare and very dangerous condition. All that can be said is to repeat the statement that in the absence of any other credible explanation the most likely basis of both idiopathic and drug-induced bone marrow failure is auto-immunity.

There is another example of aplastic anaemia of immunological interest which is associated with thymic tumour, but this is best left until the nature of myasthenia gravis is discussed on p. 168.

Auto-immune haemophilia

Another interesting blood constituent which it is convenient to mention here although it is not cellular is clotting factor VIII, genetic absence of which is responsible for haemophilia. Acquired haemophilia is a rare condition usually seen in elderly people and associated with IgG auto-antibody against factor VIII. Like the better-known disease it is associated with excessive bleeding after minor trauma. It is an interesting comment on the capacity of the body to handle difficulties in the area of immunological tolerance that Shulman records that three of thirteen cases recovered spontaneously.

CHAPTER 10

Generalized auto-immune diseases

SLE (SYSTEMIC LUPUS ERYTHEMATOSUS)

In the days before auto-immune disease was thought of and when cortisone and the other cortico-steroid drugs were still in the future, physicians had recognized a rare, acutely fatal disease of young women, characterized by fever, a bright facial rash, and a variety of visceral symptoms, with death usually coming from renal failure. The rash had some resemblance to lupus vulgaris (tuberculosis of the skin) and the disease was known as disseminated or systemic lupus erythematosus (SLE). For a long time there was a suspicion that it was a form of tuberculosis, but the bacillus was never really incriminated. If we demand an extrinsic cause for every disease, then the etiology of SLE is still unknown; but the presence of an extraordinary range of antibodies against antigens present in every cell, and rather compelling evidence that antigen–antibody complexes in the blood are concerned in the fatal kidney disease, make SLE the most outstandingly auto-immune of all human diseases.

For the last twenty years SLE has been diagnosed essentially on the basis of a single rather extraordinary serological test. Hargreaves found in 1948 that preparations of bone marrow cells from cases of SLE showed appearances which he and his collaborators called 'LE cells'. These were polymorphonuclear leucocytes containing a large, structureless, basophil-staining inclusion. It was soon found that if blood from an SLE patient was allowed to stand for an hour before being stained, similar cells could be found. Various techniques are available, but all depend on minor damage to a proportion of leucocytes in the presence of 'an antibody' in the serum. This LE factor is an IgG which is reactive with nuclear components. It enters and accumulates in the nucleus which loses its structure, swells, and is extruded from the cytoplasm, to be phagocytosed, if opportunity offers, by some polymorphonuclear cell in the neighbourhood.

Once the LE-cell test became available, it has remained the chief positive criterion for a diagnosis of SLE. Nothing in medicine is ever wholly consistent and there are patients with a positive LE-cell test who have a condition such as rheumatoid arthritis or chronic hepatitis and none of the usual signs and symptoms of SLE. Very rarely a typical case of SLE shows a negative test. In practice no physician feels happy in diagnosing SLE unless he obtains support from the laboratory in the form of an unequivocal LE-cell test. Conversely, if a patient with unusual symptoms has a positive test, she (or more rarely he) will be diagnosed probably correctly as SLE.

With the LE-cell test as the central diagnostic feature, SLE has changed from a rare disease of almost uniformly fatal outcome to a fairly common condition whose chief characteristic is intense variability in its manifestations from patient to patient and in the same patient from time to time. The commoner clinical features are: (*a*) 80–90 per cent of the cases are in females, with a peak in the young adult range of ages; (*b*) fever, facial rash, and some arthritis are common; (*c*) there is nearly always some functional damage to the kidney and death is usually due to renal failure; (*d*) in less regular fashion almost any organ of the body can be symptomatically affected. Haemolytic anaemia or thrombocytopenic purpura may occur; psychiatric disturbance or convulsions, effusion into pleural or pericardial cavities, myocarditis, valvular lesions, and chronic hepatitis may all be encountered.

From the point of view of understanding the nature of SLE, the heterogeneity of the signs and symptoms is probably just as important as the diversity of antibodies that may be produced. Much of the scientific interest in SLE has centred on the study of the many types of antibody that may be found, but it should be emphasized that there is little real evidence that the antibodies in any sense *cause* the disease. Current opinion is almost unanimous, however, that the renal lesions which are responsible for most of the deaths are due to damage by antigen–antibody complexes to the glomerular basement membrane. Haemolytic anaemia and thrombocytopenic purpura are not uncommon aspects or complications of the disease, and since they may also be seen in new-born children of mothers with SLE we can be confident that they are a fairly direct result of IgG auto-antibody action. It is still possible, however, that much of the damage is due to auto-immune T-cells. Little work has been done in this field and one can only surmise from a variety of indirect indications that their immune patterns are of the same range and diversity as the antibodies.

The abnormal antibodies

Most of the reacting factors in SLE sera have been shown to be immunoglobulin (predominantly IgG) and there is no reason to speak of them other than as antibodies. In any typical case of the disease there will be a quantitative excess of immunoglobulin and a variable range of antibodies, whose number will depend largely on the refinement of the techniques used to demonstrate them. The two standard clinical tests are for LE-cells, as described earlier, and for antinuclear factor (ANF) recognized by indirect fluorescent antibody techniques. Both probably detect mixtures of antibodies reacting with a variety of antigenic determinants in nuclei. From the theoretical angle the most important auto-antigen in SLE is DNA. Detailed study of highly reactive SLE sera with single- and double-stranded DNA combined with inhibition tests using various oligonucleotides indicates that a wide variety of sites on DNA, and particularly on denatured DNA, can serve as antigenic determinants. DNA of any origin will serve as antigen in these reactions and it underlines the intensely 'forbidden' character of such reactions that DNA, except under quite unusual conditions (see below), is quite non-immunogenic in any experimental mammal. This refers to DNA from eukaryotic organisms and bacteria. The exception that DNA from bacteriophages T2 or T4 is antigenic in the rabbit merely underlines this point, since phage DNA differs sharply in chemical structure from mammalian DNA by its content of hydroxymethyl cytosine and glucosyl (replacing some of the deoxyribosyl groups). It is therefore 'foreign' to the rabbit.

In addition to antibodies reactive with nucleic acid, there is a variety of antibodies active against intact nucleoprotein, histones, and a soluble nuclear derivative which seems to have a polysaccharide antigenic determinant. Amongst other SLE serum changes which can be ascribed to antibodies one finds positive reactions to Gajdusek and Mackay's auto-immune complement fixation test using human liver or kidney extracts and 'biological false positives' to Wassermann reagents (cardiolipin).

By no means every reactive serum shows all the types of antibodies that I have mentioned. Different patients show distinct patterns of reactivity and some positive reactions may be found in individuals who could not be suspected of suffering from SLE. Another point of interest is that patients with SLE (who not infrequently are recipients of blood transfusions) are much more prone than normal individuals to produce rare antibodies against some of the less conspicuous antigens of the red cell surface. One suspects that many other antibodies would be found in SLE sera by anyone with a new approach to human genetic polymorphisms.

It would be of very great interest to follow the development of antibodies in a typical case of SLE from before the first appearance of symptoms and it is possible that such an opportunity could be seized in clinics interested in the inheritance of auto-immune disease. There are records that a biological false positive Wassermann reaction or a raised level of gammaglobulin has preceded SLE and these could be used to screen apparently healthy members of families showing an unusual frequency of auto-immune manifestations. In the absence of detailed serial studies one can only try to deduce from the pattern of antibodies in a full-blown case the nature of the immunopathy that they reveal.

In view of the probability that auto-immune T-immunocytes play a significant role in SLE, it is unfortunate that almost nothing is known of their status in patients with the typical disease. Holman (1965) mentions that an intradermal injection of the patient's own leucocytes or a simple extract from these into her skin will usually produce a definite reaction of delayed hypersensitivity type. This presumably indicates that there are in the body specific sub-populations of T-immunocytes perhaps responsive with as large a range of 'auto' antigenic determinants as is reactive with the antibodies. For the time being, however, only the antibody findings offer any relevant basis for discussion.

Drug-induced SLE

There are two drugs, hydralazine and procainamide, which can on prolonged administration produce a clinical picture indistinguishable from a minor case of SLE. The use of hydralizine in medicine is now very limited and most of recent interest is concentrated on procainamide, which is a drug widely prescribed for the control of cardiac irregularity. Amongst persons receiving the drug for prolonged periods, up to 75 per cent may show some serological anomaly and considerable numbers show clinical changes resembling SLE. In a series of sixty-one cases the symptoms were always below the intensity of typical SLE but included fever, pleurisy, and arthritis. There was, however, no evidence of kidney involvement, no lymph node enlargement, and no cerebral symptoms. In general, the diagnosis was made on the basis of a positive LE-cell test and 94 per cent of those accepted were positive.

Most of the patients were people over 40 who had been receiving 1–4 g daily of the drug. Symptoms usually disappeared within two weeks of discontinuing the drug, but the positive serological reactions persisted for some weeks longer.

Immunopathology

A severe fatal case of SLE is the prototype of full-blown auto-immune disease and its correct interpretation would certainly lead to a general enlightenment over the whole field of auto-immunity. No one has, however, yet produced a comprehensive account of the genetic and immunological processes at work. Having regard to the interpretation of the NZB condition in an earlier chapter, four aspects of SLE need to be looked at critically. First, the genetic background; second, the inferences to be drawn from the nature of the antibodies present; third, the possibility that what was called immunological vigour in the New Zealand mice may play a part; and fourth, any evidence as to the major locus where proliferation of auto-immunocytes takes place, cf. the spleen in NZB.

1. Much has been written about genetic influence on the disease, based mainly on the search for possibly related conditions in near relatives of patients with SLE. Undoubtedly there is an excess of chronic illness of rather heterogeneous character in such families. The most striking instance was in a family described by Leonhardt where, of 14 siblings, 3 had SLE and 5 showed hypergammaglobulinaemia. Next to hypergammaglobulinaemia, the presence of auto-immune-type serological reactions, such as a positive ANF test without symptoms, was the commonest finding. Rheumatoid arthritis, thymoma, thrombocytopenic purpura, and acquired agammaglobulinaemia have also been noted amongst relatives. Quite obviously predisposition to SLE is far from being genetically simple, and equally obviously there is very little information that is relevant to the nature of either the germinal or the somatic genetic defects which must coincide before SLE is initiated.

Burch and Rowell's (1970) last analysis of the age and sex incidence of SLE is dominated by their finding that the sex ratio is curiously different as between America (M:F = 1:8) and the Netherlands (1:2). In an earlier discussion they concluded that the genetic component involved three X-linked alleles. Autosomal factors are also involved in the polygenic predisposition. The Netherlands result requires some modification in regard to the X-linked genes, but the detailed argument is irrelevant as no firm conclusion has been reached. At least we can conclude that a polygenic predisposition is concerned with a variable and sometimes gross bias to the female.

The age-specific initiation rates for SLE indicate that 'one mutation in a single stem cell in each of three distinctive sets of stem cells leads to the growth of three forbidden clones'.

2. When one looks at the serological findings in SLE it is evident at once that here there can be no question of a monoclonal condition. Clearly there are many different antibodies concerned. In addition it is known that antinuclear factors in SLE sera may be IgG, IgM, or IgA and that tests of the antibody adsorbed on to reactive nuclei always show that both γ and μ chains are present. The conspicuous presence of antinuclear and anti-DNA antibodies must be given full weight, particularly the multiplicity of nuclear antigens or antigenic determinants which can be defined with SLE sera. The general pattern of antibodies found differs rather sharply from that found amongst the localized auto-immune diseases. There are intermediate conditions such as active chronic hepatitis, but it is hard to avoid feeling that in SLE there is an immunopathological process dominating the situation which becomes much less evident in the localized auto-immune diseases.

3. For obvious reasons no systematic studies on the immune responses of SLE patients to foreign antigens have been made and evidence of anything equivalent to 'immunological vigour' must be sought from indirect indications. Perhaps the most important has already been mentioned; the undue frequency with which SLE patients who have been transfused produce the unusual or unique antibodies that are the joy of an academic haematologist. In normal individuals such findings are very much rarer. It is possible, too, that the characteristic high level of circulating immunoglobulin can also be a manifestation of immunological vigour in the sense that all types of antibody production reach an equilibrium level higher than normal. If we conclude tentatively that this evidence for immunological vigour is admissible, the quality must be a genetic one and may well represent one of the 'genes' that Burch postulates.

4. There was good evidence that the spleen played almost the sole role in the appearance of plaque-forming cells and their progenitors in NZB mice. In SLE there is no such direct evidence, and what hints there are point to a general involvement of the whole lymphoid system. The nature of the antibodies produced suggests that immunocyte proliferation is likely to be occurring in regions where nuclei are present in various stages of disintegration. This immediately suggests that it is worth exploring the role of regions of active lymphocytic proliferation such as the thymic cortex or germinal centres in lymph nodes and spleen. It is characteristic of these regions that in addition to proliferation there is death of considerable numbers of lymphocytes, with pyknosis and degeneration of nuclei. The hypothesis might be tested that in this particular environment normal circumstances ensure that contact of newly born, i.e. newly differentiated, immunocytes with a corresponding self-antigen results in their elimination. It is, however, an environment liable to differ from the normal either directly by inheritance or particularly in some genotypes as a result of modification by metabolic changes or certain drugs, so that contact of self-antigenic determinant and reactive immunocyte results not infrequently in a proliferative rather than destructive stimulus. Once this happened there would be possibilities of autocatalytic damage, particularly in the thymus, where most or all of the proliferating auto-immunocytes would be of the T series. One would expect a complex situation which might well include (*a*) stress atrophy of the cortex, (*b*) proliferation of thymic epithelial cells, (*c*) appearance of germinal centres, and (*d*) plasma cells and mast cells in increased numbers. These are what have been found in a thymus removed from a girl with early SLE. On the assumption that the early stages of such disorganization of thymic function will accentuate the switch from destruction to proliferation of newly differentiated cells with receptors tuned to self-antigens, we could well expect the spread of similar dysfunction to the other lymphoid tissues of the body. The failure of thymectomy in the case mentioned above to improve the condition would fit with this assumption. Once large numbers of auto-immune cells particularly capable of reacting with damaged lymphoid cells are in existence it is obvious that every lymphocytic function will be liable to fall into chaos. This is a phrase which is perhaps appropriate to the picture presented by a severe case of SLE.

A further point worth consideration is the often acute onset of SLE in a person previously healthy. This tends to be ascribed to a minor infection, use of a drug, or some psychosocial trauma. None of these sounds particularly convincing, yet there is strong reason to suspect that some 'trigger' has in fact set a self-intensifying autocatalytic process in train. It is in the early stages of that process that we might find a revealing sequence of immunological changes. Until such data are available, only guesses are possible. The results with procainamide are important in indicating that processes resembling low-grade SLE can be initiated by the drug in persons who are certainly *not* genetically predisposed to the disease. This suggests that predisposition plus a metabolic change in some way related to the action of procainamide allows an autocatalytic accentuation of the same process once it has been set in motion. The possibility that the hypothetical metabolic process was initiated in the thymic cortex is a mere guess, but it seems not unreasonable in view of the extreme susceptibility of thymocytes to undergo destruction under almost any type of severe stress.

Relatively few cases of SLE present the classical acutely fatal picture and any interpretation must be compatible with the existence of an infinitely graded range from the normal to hyperacute SLE. That range is basically an indication of the transcending complexity of the living organism and the random character of all genetic change. In every direction there is a need for multiple fail-safe controls to deal with genetic or metabolic accident, but the controls themselves are subject to similar accidents. SLE is almost certainly not a 'natural' disease entity but a rather arbitrarily defined segment of a wide range of overlapping and interrelated auto-immune conditions which includes rheumatoid arthritis and many rarer conditions. Further discussion of the pathogenesis of SLE is better deferred till these have been dealt with.

RHEUMATOID ARTHRITIS

The typical picture of rheumatoid arthritis in a middle-aged or elderly woman, with hands distorted and deviated to the ulnar side, is familiar to almost everyone. This, however, is merely a common late result of a protean disease which may begin acutely or insidiously, affect almost any pattern of joints and show wide differences in its course and in its amenability to the conventionally used therapeutic measures. There is a relatively rare but well-defined childhood form of the disease in which the general symptoms of fever and weight loss are more conspicuous than in adults. At all ages the most urgent symptoms are associated with synovitis of the joints leading to a variety of secondary local changes. There are inflammatory lesions of similar character in other synovial surfaces, bursas, tendon sheaths, etc., and subcutaneous rheumatoid nodules are common.

The problem of etiology

All pathologists are agreed that auto-immune processes are actively concerned in persisting rheumatoid arthritis, but a majority would probably express doubts about its *initiation* by auto-immune processes and remain expectant that a micro-organismal agent or group of agents will eventually be incriminated. The auto-immune interpretation is that the symptoms and pathological changes depend on the presence of auto-antibody against immunoglobulin perhaps associated with T-immunocytes of similar specificity.

Anti-immunoglobulins, the so-called rheumatoid factors, are frequently found in the serum, particularly in patients in acute and severe disease. There are various ways in which they can be detected, but they nearly always involve the use as test antigen of particulate material coated with partly denatured human immunoglobulin G. Human red cells coated with incomplete human antibody or latex particles non-specifically coated are often used. The auto-antibodies frequently react with other mammalian immunoglobulins and the most commonly used test is probably with sheep red cells coated with standard antibody from a rabbit at a level beneath that needed to provoke agglutination. Rheumatoid factor causes agglutination of any of these test cells or particles.

The term rheumatoid factor (RF) covers a highly complex situation in which anti-immunoglobulins, usually IgM but sometimes IgG, react with antigenic determinants present on IgG. As isolated, RF most commonly consists of an IgM molecule, the essential auto-antibody, loosely combined with several IgG molecules presumably functioning as antigen in an antigen–antibody complex. Detailed study uncovers many differences amongst the anti-immunoglobulins of sera from patients with rheumatoid arthritis. Apart from underlining the heterogeneity of the antibody clones which must be involved, the detail of this complexity is irrelevant in the present context.

A second type of approach depends on histological evidence that in actively involved joints it is regular to find leucocytes containing inclusions of aggregated immunoglobulin in the cytoplasm. It has also been shown that cells reactive with immunoglobulin are present in lymphoid accumulations within the joints and in germinal centres of draining lymph nodes.

On this basis it is relatively straightforward to describe the condition as an auto-immune disease in which the symptoms can be ascribed to immune reactions against IgG immunoglobulin. Yet everyone is aware that over 1 per cent of normal people have anti-IgG detectable in serum and the proportion increases with age. The great majority show no signs of rheumatoid arthritis. In older people, both the frequency of arthritis and of positive RF reactions increase with age, though not necessarily in parallel in each individual, and in the great majority of people with high-titre RF, symptoms of arthritis are present. On the other hand, in any group of patients diagnosed clinically as rheumatoid arthritis, a majority will be sero-negative to the standard tests. The most definite statement that can be made is probably that severe cases of rheumatoid arthritis with extra-articular symptoms almost always have clear signs of immunological reactivity: a high titre of rheumatoid factor, intracytoplasmic inclusions of denatured Ig, and a diminished complement titre in joint fluid.

Serological studies on rheumatoid arthritis have been concentrated on anti-immunoglobulins just as those on SLE have centred on antibodies against DNA and other nuclear components. The reasons are obvious. No immunologist interested in details of specificity cares to work with anything but a serum with a high content of the antibodies he is interested in from a full-blown case of the disease. Much less attention has been paid to any minor components in such 'specially typical' sera and even less to sera with lower titres or from less typical cases.

In view of the overlap amongst all the generalized auto-immune diseases which has already been mentioned and will call for further discussion, this clear separation is almost certainly false. Both SLE and rheumatoid arthritis, if closely enough studied, will show a fringe of other immunological abnormalities as well as those toward which attention is almost exclusively directed in the literature. In the following discussion of the significance of anti-immunoglobulins in rheumatoid arthritis, this qualification must always be kept in mind.

To account for the significance of those antibodies, there seem to be two basic etiological hypotheses:

1. That a common potential pathogen, a mycoplasma perhaps, lodges in the synovial area. As part of the normal response to an invading micro-organism, specific antibody is produced. In certain people the immunoglobulin of the antibody can serve as antigen and provoke a secondary immunological response. This results in the presence in the circulating blood of much IgM antibody, which reacts with IgG particularly when it is partially denatured. A vicious circle is initiated in which the irritant qualities of immunoglobulin complexes (IgG/IgM anti-IgG) are responsible for symptoms.

2. That rheumatoid arthritis is a primary auto-immune disease due to the appearance and proliferation of forbidden clones of immunocytes reactive with immunoglobulin as antigen. It may be necessary to postulate, in addition, some triggering mechanism, localized to joints, to set the process under way. A possible model of such a trigger is the common polyarthritis associated with an attack of rubella in an adult, and there are probably many other minor infections which might on occasion localize Ag–Ab complexes in the synovial area. In the vast majority of people they clear up in a few days or weeks.

The status of IgG, or immunoglobulins generally as auto-antigens, is not fully clarified. Undoubtedly immunoglobulin partially denatured is a much better antigen when injected into a foreign species than if care is taken to inject only soluble antigen freed of all aggregates. It is not clear whether this is because of the exposure of new antigenic determinants with partial denaturation or simply because of the physical differences between the two forms. Both aspects may be relevant. When immunoglobulin is concerned as an auto-antigen it seems rather highly probable that immunogenicity is greatly increased when it is presented in the form of antibody bound to a bacterial surface and partly denatured thereby. In subacute bacterial endocarditis there is persistent liberation of bacteria coated with antibody from the valvular lesions and an almost regular production of an antibody functionally similar to rheumatoid factor. This is not associated with arthritis and if the condition is cured by antibiotic therapy the anti-immunoglobulin disappears. Something more than the production of RF is obviously required for the development of rheumatoid arthritis; a genetic predisposition is fairly obviously one requirement.

Given the necessary genetic predisposition, and having due regard to Burch's formulations, the appearance of rheumatoid arthritis at such and such an age must be ascribed to the accumulation of sufficient numbers of auto-immunocytes and their products. Each line concerned arises in the last analysis from an inheritable change in a single cell. In essence, the immature immunocytes derived from proliferation of such a mutant, if they are going to give rise to cells producing anti-immunoglobulins, must (*a*) be capable of reacting specifically with an antigenic determinant carried on an IgG molecule and (*b*) be unduly resistant to destruction or functional inhibition as a result of specific contact. Neither the nature of the genetic change nor the phenotypic changes in the descendant cells can be expressed in other than functional terms. The only certainties are that somatic mutation is always rare and informationally random and that many different mutations may be effective. The findings from clinical serology show that the anti-IgGs, the rheumatoid factors, are highly heterogeneous and may react with a variety of antigenic determinants; there can be no unique type of mutation which alone leads to rheumatoid arthritis.

With the reservation that we are concerned with a speculative exercise on how a stochastic approach may be devised to fit the facts of rheumatoid arthritis, some further elaboration may be permissible.

We assume that among all the possible immune-receptor patterns which can emerge on differentiated immunocytes there are three (*A*, *B*, and *C*) which will react effectively with IgG partially denatured in the form of an Ag–Ab complex. In the sequence of stem cells arising from the bone marrow a certain very small proportion will be potential *A* producers. Others will similarly be predestined to produce *B* or *C*. For the next step we assume that any stem cell including *A*, *B*, or *C* is liable to a mutational change to the control-resistant condition R. There will be reasons why this is more likely to happen in persons genetically prone to rheumatoid arthritis than in others, but there is no need to speculate about these reasons here. All we need to say is that a stem cell of potentiality *A* can become A^R at any point in its history from the fertilized egg onward, but there will be no possible effect until *A* is phenotypically expressed and a cell of the clone becomes an immunocyte. However, if the A^R situation is established early in the ontogeny of a stem cell line, a number of descendant cells will be available for differentiation to immunocytes.

There are two points to be recalled from the previous discussion of immunocyte differentiation. The first is that the essential receptor or combining site is of the same basic structure for all immunocytes or antibodies of the same clonal origin and the second that the type of immunocyte to which a stem cell differentiates is determined by the local micro-environment where the process takes place. If, then, a small clone of potential A^R stem cells enters the circulation, its members may develop in more than one fashion. Some might emerge as T-cells, as IgM-producers (some capable of switch to IgG, some not), or as IgA-producers. Only one type may be able to prosper or any combination of different types.

If we go a little further and accept the indications for a genetic predisposition to auto-immune disease as valid, then there will be an abnormally high (but still probably very low in commonsense terms) likelihood that, in addition to the clone A^R, mutation will give rise to other ^{R} clones of *A*, *B*, or *C* which will have similar randomized opportunities to emerge as T-cells or immunoglobulin-producers of one or other type.

Such speculation may sound inadmissible to anyone trained primarily at a chemical level, but it is strictly analogous to any population genetics approach to the problems of evolution of species. The whole complex of defensive and homoeostatic activities of the circulating cells must be interpreted in terms of the population dynamics of the cell types concerned; and this must hold equally for any pathological deviations of the systems which may arise.

The simplest hypothesis of rheumatoid arthritis, then, is that it represents an abnormal immune response to immunoglobulins whose antigenicity has been slightly modified by forming part of an Ag–Ab complex. The actual role of the anti-immunoglobulin is still problematical. Transfusion of blood from rheumatoid arthritis patients with high titres of rheumatoid factor into volunteers had no effect whatever, and it is well known that most early cases of rheumatoid arthritis are negative to tests for RF. If one is to be consistent in assuming a primary auto-immune origin for the disease, it seems necessary to demand that the condition begins as the result of a cell-mediated (T) response against the Ig determinant. However, the point may have to be left indeterminate until at least two other alternatives have been fully assessed. The first is the possible trigger effect already mentioned of an infection like rubella, the second the possibility of a primary auto-immune attack against a tissue-specific synovial antigen. Irrespective of the primary agent, many cases will in due course develop some form of RF in the circulation. Most pathologists ascribe some damaging possibilities to the auto-antibody, but there is no unanimity about its action.

The presence of RF may have a net result of either accentuating the pathological progress or protecting against it. There is a relatively high correlation between high antibody titres and severe, 'complicated' rheumatoid arthritis. On the other hand, many persons with RF have no evidence of rheumatoid arthritis, while in agammaglobulinaemic individuals with no circulating RF and only traces of immunoglobulin arthritis with many resemblances to the rheumatoid type is very common.

The heterogeneity of rheumatoid arthritis

Variability in the manifestations of rheumatoid arthritis is proverbial. Some of the variants, when fully expressed, have specific labels but all show continuous gradings to the standard form. The more important types justifying individual mention are: Still's disease (juvenile rheumatoid arthritis); the Felty syndrome in which rheumatoid arthritis is associated with splenic enlargement and neutropenia; and systemic rheumatoid disease in which cardiac, pulmonary, or renal manifestations are conspicuous. There are two well-defined conditions (systemic lupus erythematosus (SLE) and rheumatic fever) which in 90 per cent of cases are sharply differentiable but which can in some individuals present clinical or serological manifestations of rheumatoid arthritis. Sjögren's syndrome is a form of rheumatoid arthritis which is important enough to call for a more extended discussion on p. 147. Finally, one should mention the characteristic joint involvement of rubella and of serum sickness and the rare instances in which severe rheumatoid arthritis is associated with a malignant tumour and shows remission when the tumour is removed.

Every case is to some extent individual and prognosis is notoriously difficult. Irregular remissions and exacerbations are the rule, with slow progression to deformity and crippling, but remissions may be effectively permanent at any time and elderly 'burnt-out' cases with gross distortion of the hands but no other symptoms are often seen. Any interpretation of the etiology of rheumatoid arthritis must be flexible enough to cover this immense range of variability. This is in fact the chief or only justification for basing the etiology on random mutations in single cells.

Equally relevant and equally difficult to fit into a tidy pattern is the distribution of positive RF reactions in relation to other disease conditions. Adequate testing will often show a proportion of transient positive reactions after almost any situation which calls for an antibody response, particularly when it is of a chronic character. Subacute bacterial endocarditis, already mentioned, and chronic bronchitis are the classic examples. Macroglobulinaemia in the form associated with purpura of the legs and usually polyclonal in character shows nearly 100 per cent of positive RF reactions, and a considerable proportion of monoclonal paraproteinaemias, whether IgM or IgG, show RF character. As might perhaps be expected, most such sera show precipitation of immunoglobulin aggregates when stored in the cold and are classed clinically as cryoglobulinaemias.

Age incidence of rheumatoid arthritis and other joint affections

Burch's first studies on the age incidence of auto-immune disease were made on Lawrence's data for inflammatory polyarthritis, i.e. one clinical aspect of the general complex, rheumatoid arthritis. His conclusions were that quantitative data on age, sex, and grading (1–4) of intensity of disease could be interpreted in terms of (1) an approximate 50 per cent of susceptibility (genetic), (2) a process by which somatic mutation occurred in stem cells of the lymphoid series, allowing emergence of forbidden arthritogenic clones at a rate constant throughout adult life, (3) a probability of somatic mutation twice as high in females as in males, (4) a relation between the intensity of disease and the number of independent somatic mutations arising.

In a subsequent discussion Burch separates the three factors observable in 'rheumatoid arthritis' as inflammatory polyarthritis, erosive arthritis radiologically visible, and positive serological tests for rheumatoid factor. He finds that the age incidence for rheumatoid arthritis as defined by the American Rheumatism Association is not capable of analysis by his methods. The entities erosive arthritis, inflammatory arthritis, ankylosing spondylitis, and osteo-arthrosis, however, all give age- and sex-specific prevalence curves which can be interpreted to give values for (*a*) the proportion genetically predisposed, (*b*) the number of somatic mutations needed to initiate a given grade of disease, (*c*) the rate

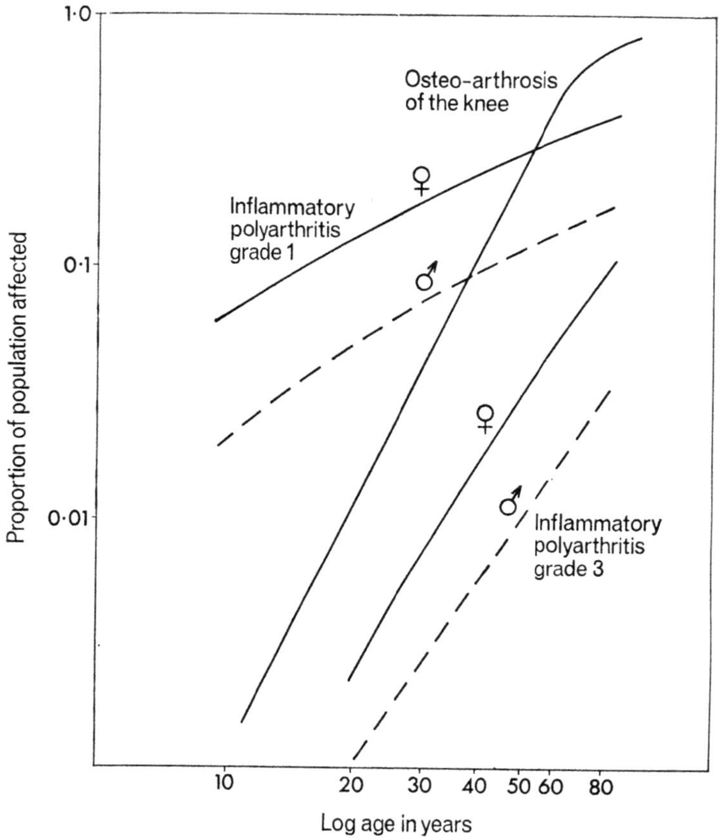

FIG. 20. To illustrate the age-specific prevalence of arthritic conditions in man, as plotted by Burch's method. These are simplified curves from Burch (1968) showing the proportion of the population with signs of: (1) Inflammatory polyarthritis of mild (grade 1) and severe (grade 3) degree in males and females. (2) Osteo-arthrosis of the knee joint. Both scales are logarithmic. (J. J. R. Duthie and W. R. M. Alexander (eds), *Rheumatic Diseases*, Medical Monograph 3, Edinburgh University Press, 1968.)

constant for clone initiation, and (*d*) the latent period between clone initiation and recognition of symptoms.

Subject to earlier qualifications as to the limitations of stochastic mathematical analysis of highly complex biological situations, some points of interest from Burch's calculations may be mentioned.

Everyone is potentially susceptible to osteo-arthritis and probably to erosive arthritis, but only 50 per cent of people to inflammatory polyarthritis and 0·1 per cent to ankylosing spondylitis. Three or four initiating somatic mutations are required for clinically evident disease in all except inflammatory polyarthritis, where one somatic mutation only is needed for grade 1 disease.

To indicate the type of age incidence seen in the subacute to chronic joint conditions, I have combined in Fig. 20 simplified data in the form of smoothed curves for inflammatory polyarthritis grade 1 and grade 3 male and female, and for arthrosis of the knee. In each the absolute age prevalence is shown; it approaches 100 per cent in arthrosis and 50 per cent in inflammatory polyarthritis. Ankylosing spondylitis and other rarer forms provide similar curves at a lower level of incidence. The curves are only approximately accurate, but they do show the striking differences within this group of diseases and the possibilities of stochastic analysis.

The very simple straight line for osteo-arthrosis curving off only at old age as it approaches the asymptotic 100 per cent is worthy of some comment. This curve for arthrosis of the knee is quite similar in form to those constructed for the same type of disease in other joints such as the small joints of hand and foot. It is of interest, however, that only in the results for proximal interphalangeal joints is there a significant difference between the sexes, the female incidence being twice as high at each age. The equation is of similar form, $Pt = 1 - e^{-kt^4}$, for all, with k varying from one set of joints to another. According to Burch's interpretation, this indicates that four mutational events occurring sequentially in at least one stem cell are needed. As soon as the necessary fourth mutation has been achieved the cell can initiate a process leading to grade 2 lesions in ten years, to grade 3 lesions in twenty-six years. As yet there are no other indications that osteo-arthrosis is an auto-immune disease in any ordinary sense; a common synonym is degenerative arthropathy and it is commonly regarded as an aspect of the ageing process. The possibility that this and similar degenerative changes may be legitimately equated with auto-immune processes is discussed in Chapter 15.

Sjögren's syndrome and other conditions

In a proportion of cases with otherwise typical rheumatoid arthritis there are additional symptoms, dry eyes (kerato-conjunctivitis sicca) and dry mouth (xerostomia), which result from cellular infiltration of the lacrimal and salivary glands respectively. In some there is visible swelling of the parotid glands. Recently attention has been drawn to the occurrence of renal tubular acidosis in some patients with Sjögren's syndrome with an associated lymphocytic and plasma cell infiltration of interstitial spaces in the kidney. The infiltration is basically similar to that in lacrimal and salivary glands (Talal, 1971).

Such patterns of organ infiltration are usually associated with rheumatoid arthritis, but Boyle and Buchanan point out that there are nearly as many cases where the same types of infiltration are seen with SLE. In their view the infiltrative lesions with their functional symptoms may be associated with any one of the generalized auto-immune conditions which have also been known as collagen diseases or connective tissue diseases. They comprise rheumatoid arthritis, SLE, progresssive systemic sclerosis (or scleroderma), polymyositis, dermatomyositis, and polyarteritis nodosa. Only a brief account of the clinical and immunological characteristics of these conditions seems to be called for, particularly as the clinical pictures are highly variable and often include features of more than one of the conventional types. The diagnosis in fact is simply related to the organ or tissue which seems to be most conspicuously involved.

Polymyositis and dermatomyositis involve muscle and the main symptom is muscular weakness, mainly involving the proximal limb muscles but with difficulty in swallowing not uncommon. Sections of affected muscles show varying degrees of lymphocytic and plasma cell infiltration.

In dermatomyositis and progressive systemic sclerosis the skin is extensively involved. In dermatomyositis muscle changes are also present, and in systemic sclerosis a variety of visceral lesions may be present as well as the skin condition. A considerable proportion of cases of dermatomyositis are associated with the presence of a malignant tumour somewhere in the body.

Some involvement of arteries and arterioles can be seen in any disease of the group, but in periarteritis nodosa the main pathological change takes the form of numerous foci of inflammatory or necrotic arteritis.

The mode of onset and severity of these conditions are all variable, but, in general, treatment with adequate doses of corticosteroids will control initial acute symptoms in all of them although rarely providing long continued control. From the therapeutic angle they are all unrewarding.

Discussion and summary

It is the heterogeneity of the clinical material and the virtual impossibility of sorting cases into a small number of categories that convinces me of the relevance and the complexity of interacting somatic mutational and control processes. I have earlier expressed a scepticism about Burch's precise formulation of the need for so many sequential or concurrent somatic mutational episodes to give the observed specific age incidence of an auto-immune disease. I do not dispute the likelihood that several events must happen at random to produce a certain pattern of disease, but I cannot conceive that a precise specification of the number and type of mutations can ever be anything better than an 'as if' exercise. Even so, it can be highly valuable in providing a qualitative interpretation of the complexities of this group of 'collagen diseases'. In the next page or two I have used a non-mathematical recasting of several of Burch's ideas to attempt an interpretation of the diversity of disease that we have discussed in this chapter.

There is still no accepted hypothesis to account for the overlap amongst SLE, rheumatoid arthritis, systemic sclerosis, dermatomyositis, and polyarteritis nodosa nor for the manifest similarities in another sense of the erosive arthritis of the rheumatoid arthritis complex, spinal ankylosis, and osteo-arthrosis. However, if one accepts both the forbidden clone concept and Burch's contention that for a forbidden clone to emerge several mutations (or more broadly rare and random events) must occur, a relatively satisfying solution can be envisaged.

At an earlier stage I have indicated that in some species at least a mutation which will eventually result in a certain phenotypic expression in a particular tissue can occur at any stage in the ancestry of the cell line concerned. It can be a dominant mutation in the germ cell line or it can occur at any stage in the cell line leading from the fertilized ovum to the immediate precursor of the cells showing the phenotypic change. The proportion of cells showing the change will clearly be 100 per cent if the responsible mutation is germinal and progressively less and less as the time of somatic mutation becomes further and further removed from the first segmentation division of the zygote.

When the stem lines from which immunocytes are derived are involved in somatic mutations relevant to the development of auto-immune qualities, some quite important implications arise. We can follow Jerne in assuming that the newly formed genome of the zygote has a rather small number of immediate potentialities for immune patterns. Diversification from each of these genetically acquired patterns takes place in embryonic and post-natal life by still unknown processes equivalent in result to somatic mutation and selection. By hypothesis, the process is going on from some early stage of differentiation to a much later stage at which phenotypic restriction becomes operative and the immune pattern characteristic of subsequent descendants is fixed. Any somatic mutation which when phenotypically expressed renders a descendant immunocyte resistant to the normal process of control and elimination will necessarily be transmitted to all descendant clones derived from the cell line subsequent to the occurrence of the mutation. A variety of 'families' of forbidden clones thus becomes possible. In the limit *all* immunocytes would be involved if the mutation was of germinal origin or took place immediately after fusion of the male and female nuclei. If it occurred at any subsequent stage, it would involve only those lines stemming from the mutant cell. Assuming that the mutation to resistance occurred at a relatively early stage these could continue immune pattern diversification so that an extensive range of immune patterns reactive with self-components could be involved. If one assumes that three steps are needed before the full resistance to control is developed and that for at least one or possibly two a 'phenocopy' of a somatic genetic change can be produced by drug action or metabolic change, a wide diversity of result becomes possible. It will still hold, however, that the earlier the relevant mutations arise the wider will be the effect. The diversity and variable intensity of the manifestations of SLE could well be referred to the stage in stem cell development when the different relevant factors, genetic (in the normal sense), somatic mutational, metabolic, or pharmacological came into play.

An approach of this general character would fit the picture presented by the multiplicity of antibodies found in SLE, the overlap between differently named auto-immune diseases and the fact that some auto-immune conditions are limited to one target organ without even corresponding auto-antibody while others show every possible stage of increasing diversity of pathogenic activity and antibody till we reach the full-blown, rapidly fatal case of SLE.

It is at least clear that any interpretation of SLE and the overlapping 'collagen' diseases must probably be almost as complex as the clinical manifestations of the disease themselves. The factors which

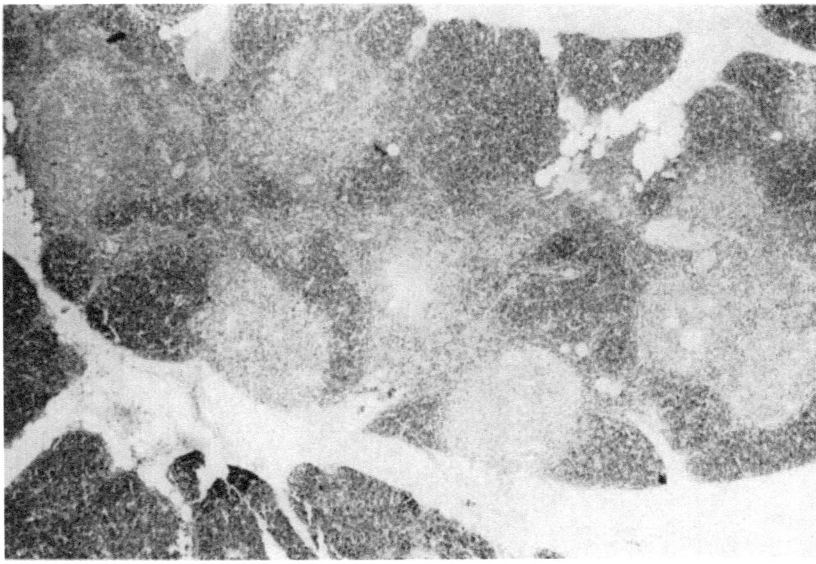

A

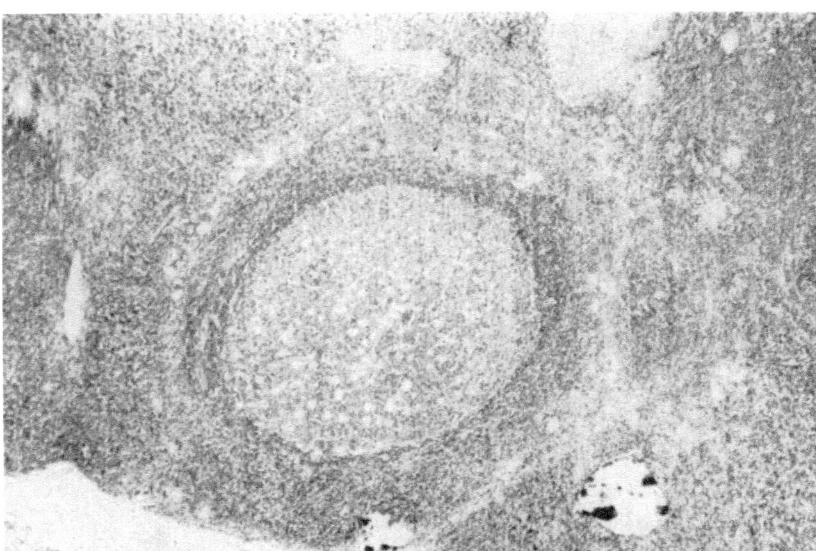

B

PLATE 4. Germinal centres in the thymus of a patient with myasthenia gravis. *a*. Low power showing several germinal centres. *b*. Higher power showing rather pale staining cells of the germinal centre with narrow rim of close-packed dark staining small lymphocytes.

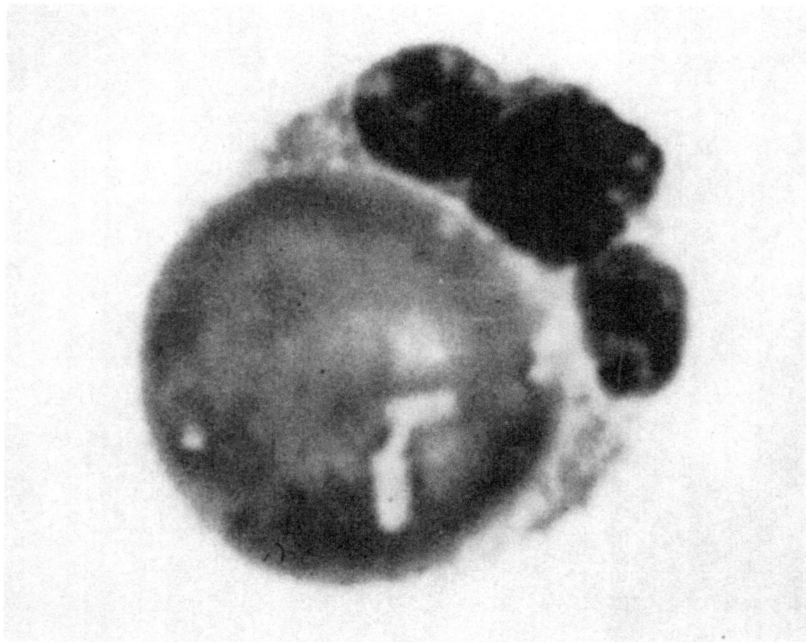

PLATE 2. An LE cell from a case of SLE. The round, almost featureless mass is a swollen nucleus ingested by a polymorphonuclear leucocyte whose own nucleus is seen at the side. (Mackay and Burnet, 1963.)

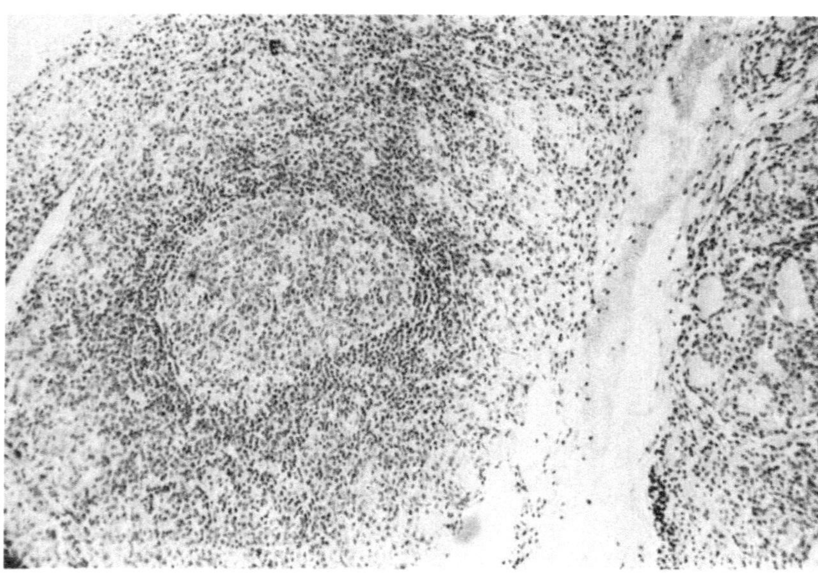

PLATE 3. Germinal centre in thyroid gland of a patient with Hashimoto's thyroiditis. There is also heavy diffuse infiltration of lymphocytes throughout the gland.

have been discussed and regarded as relevant can be enumerated as follows:

1. Genetic factors are important, including those determining the predominantly female incidence. It is a polygenic condition not yet susceptible to detailed analysis.

2. 'Immunological vigour' may be one component of the genetically controlled background.

3. The characteristic age and sex incidence implies a series of somatic mutational changes. It may be expressing virtually the same idea to say that active auto-immune disease only emerges when the several components of a fail-safe system of control are overcome.

4. The variety of auto-antibodies suggests that the forbidden clones responsible are stimulated to proliferate in lymphoid tissue where cells are actively multiplying and where some of them are undergoing autolysis.

5. Some of the mutational changes needed can be imitated by the effect of certain drugs or metabolites on the micro-environment.

Taken together, these points offer an interpretation which is based, as any interpretation must be, on the accepted theoretical basis of immunology, which introduces no unrelated concept such as an undiscovered virus, and which is concordant with the main clinical features of SLE, its characteristic age and sex incidence and its great variability of expression in symptoms, course and duration, pathological changes and, above all, in the anomalous immunological qualities of the blood serum.

CHAPTER 11

Localized auto-immune diseases

The third major grouping of auto-immune disease comprises those conditions which wholly or predominantly involve a single organ or tissue. There are many forms of localized auto-immune disease with thyroid, gastric mucosa, and adrenal as the sites for some of the better-studied examples. As in other fields, there is no universally acceptable interpretation of the conditions to be discussed in this chapter. No one questions that all present important immunopathological aspects, but it can usually be claimed that these are the secondary consequences of pathological changes in the organ induced by some primary etiological agent. This suggests that it may be useful to precede discussion of the various local conditions with a brief consideration at a general level.

Irrespective of any questions of etiology it is obvious to every physician that there are a number of diseases which arise at some more or less well-defined age and involve an organ or other functional entity which was known to be functioning normally up to the time of onset. Hyperthyroidism, idiopathic Addison's disease of the adrenals, acromegaly, myasthenia gravis may be taken as examples of such diseases where we can clearly exclude an infectious or toxic agent from outside. Looked at from first principles, there are not a great number of ways by which a genetically normal organ can develop localized disease confined to the organ. The possibilities are:

1. It may be invaded secondarily by micro-organisms or malignant cells that have been responsible for or been generated by primary disease somewhere else in the body.

2. Hormonal over- or under-stimulation may induce functional change that is sufficiently abnormal to rank as disease.

3. A tumour may arise from a single cell in the organ and grow destructively.

4. An auto-immune process mediated by antibody or T-cells is directed against an antigenic determinant characteristic of the organ.

Conditions coming under the first of these headings will usually be recognized as secondary to the primary disease in the ordinary course of clinical examination and do not call for further discussion here.

The other three conditions, however, have a common feature that is highly relevant to our general theme. In one way or another, somatic mutation plays a significant role in the disease process, whether this is primarily malignant or auto-immune. This holds as much for (2) as for (3) and (4). Hormonal over- or under-stimulation will be secondary to change in another endocrine organ, usually the pituitary. The process responsible for *that* abnormality is almost limited to neoplastic change or auto-immune attack. Irrespective of whatever ideas one may hold about the process of carcinogenesis, the emergent tumour is initially a clone of mutant cells, the modification in the initiating cell being of the quality of a somatic mutation. Finally, any auto-immune process, according to the view that has been consistently adopted in this book, must be initiated by a single or more probably a sequence of somatic mutations in a stem cell line ancestral to immunocytes.

In other words, this is a claim that all pathological processes not due to the impact of the environment which arise in specific organs that have previously been genetically normal arise directly or indirectly from somatic genetic changes. There are almost certainly rare exceptions, but the rule is one that I believe is salutary for the clarification of thought on etiological problems.

Auto-immune disease of the thyroid

The concepts of localized auto-immune disease have been built up very largely in relation to thyroid disease. Hashimoto's disease is the most common forerunner of myxoedema and remains the classical example of infiltrative auto-immune disease with progressive functional deterioration of the organ. The possibility of producing a histologically similar condition in experimental animals by immunization with homologous or even autologous thyroid extracts in Freund's complete adjuvant acted as a further stimulus to its study. Around 1964 still further interest in thyroid immunity was evoked by the discovery that the so-called long-acting thyroid stimulator (LATS) was not, as had been thought, a modified or genetically anomalous thyroid-stimulating hormone (TSH) from the pituitary but an immunoglobulin G, and therefore, by implication, an auto-antibody. It is far from being proven that the manifestations of thyrotoxicosis result from stimulation of the gland by the auto-antibody LATS, but the relationship does make it extremely probable that toxic goitre is as much an auto-immune disease as Hashimoto's disease or myxoedema.

Studies of human sera from Hashimoto's disease and other thyroid diseases have revealed many ways by which thyroid-specific antibodies can be detected. There seem to be at least three well-defined types of antigenic determinants:

1. Thyroglobulin antibody can be detected by precipitation, complement fixation, tanned red cell agglutination, and fluorescent staining which shows concentration of the antigen in the colloid of thyroid vesicles.
2. Antibody to a microsomal cytoplasmic component can be shown by complement fixation and fluorescent techniques. It is also this antibody which is responsible for cytocidal action on thyroid cells in culture.
3. A second colloid antigen (CA2), possibly a thyroid protease, is detectable by some antisera from Hashimoto patients.

It is still uncertain whether any of these antibodies should be regarded as in any sense responsible for actual thyroid damage.

The fourth thyroid auto-antibody, LATS, already referred to in relation to exophthalmic (toxic) goitre, is detected by a rather elaborate functional test *in vivo*. The agent can be absorbed from serum by thyroid tissue and is fixed on the microsomal fraction.

There is little that is relevant to the possible role of auto-immune T-cells in thyroid disease. Skin reactions of delayed hypersensitivity type may result from intradermal injection of thyroid extracts in Hashimoto patients. Immunization of guinea-pigs with homologous thyroid tissue in FCA gives a proportion of thyroiditis with round cell infiltration. Animals may also develop skin reactivity or complement fixing antibody and there is a much closer correlation of thyroiditis with delayed hypersensitivity than with antibody production.

Thyrotoxicosis

In classical Graves's disease with a functionally hyperactive thyroid the main features are enlarged, highly vascular thyroid, tremor, increased basal metabolic rate, and protruding (exophthalmic) eyes. There is a wide range of ages amongst patients, but there is a predominance of cases in young adult women of much the same type as is seen in SLE.

In a study of age-specific incidence, using Burch's approach, a Canadian group found a typical 'auto-immune' graph giving best fit with an r value of 3. In other words, it behaves as if three independent somatic mutations were required. It appears to be at least a good working hypothesis that thyrotoxicosis is a primary auto-immune disease.

Positive support for the hypothesis can be sought from the following:

1. Antibodies against thyroglobulin and reacting by complement fixation are frequently present.

2. Many toxic thyroids removed surgically show lymphocytic infiltration. There is a correlation between the amount of infiltration and the likelihood of positive serological reactions.

3. The heavier the cellular infiltration, the more likely the patient was to show signs of inadequate thyroid function after subtotal thyroidectomy.

4. A proportion of cases show LATS antibody and the proportion becomes virtually 100 per cent in individuals with both well-marked exophthalmos and pretibial oedema.

None of this is at all decisive; there are cases of typical hyperthyroidism which show no serological reactions and only minimal cellular infiltration. Conversely, there are very large numbers of persons with a variety of other conditions or apparently healthy who also show thyroid antibodies. Another pointer against an auto-immune process may be the fact that probably not more than 10 per cent of thyrotoxicosis cases go on to Hashimoto's disease and myxoedema.

Certainly if it is an auto-immune disease thyrotoxicosis has some unique features, and this may be a partial justification for looking closely at LATS which, as an antibody, is equally unique. LATS is detected by its power to increase iodine metabolism in the thyroid of mice and could be expected, if it were infused steadily into a normal human being, to produce symptoms of thyrotoxicosis. This has been rather frequently done as an experiment of nature when women are actively thyrotoxic with circulating LATS in the later stages of pregnancy. A number of reports of congenital thyrotoxicosis in such infants have been reported; in a group of four babies reported by Hoffmann *et al.*, all showed LATS in the blood. The antibody is IgG, a molecule small enough to pass readily across the placenta; the normal TSH does not do so. In another series of infants born with thyrotoxicosis, all had lost all symptoms by 3 months. It is hard to find any reason against accepting maternal LATS as responsible for the symptoms in the infants. With its progressive removal with the rest of the maternal IgG in the first few months the disappearance of symptoms is only to be expected.

The most obvious hypothesis, though as far as I know it has not been experimentally tested, is that by some quirk of peptide chemistry the combining site of the LATS antibody sufficiently resembles the effector configuration of TSH to unite with the same receptors on the surface of thyroid cells. This is consistent with the experimental finding that the response to TSH and LATS is additive and that a similar prolonged response can be obtained when the short half-life in the body of TSH is countered by giving it in repeated small doses.

Hashimoto's disease

There are many minor variants of subacute thyroiditis with forms that merge on one side with thyrotoxicosis, including nodular toxic forms, and on the other with myxoedema. The diagnosis of Hashimoto's disease is based primarily on the histology (lymphocytic infiltration often with germinal centres), the presence of thyroid auto-antibodies, and the absence of evidence of thyroid hyperactivity. Doniach *et al.* divided 84 cases of Hashimoto's disease into: classical Hashimoto's disease 58, mild lymphocytic thyroiditis 11, thyroiditis superimposed on Graves's disease 10, and primary myxoedema 5. In some instances Hashimoto's disease remains stable for long periods, but in general there is progressive deficiency of thyroid function, and it is likely that all or most cases of myxoedema represent the end result of an auto-immune process that at some stage would be diagnosable as Hashimoto's disease.

Much information is available about antibodies in these cases, but very little about cell-mediated immunity, which is almost certainly more important. The chief interest of the antibody studies is in relation to the question of genetic susceptibility to local auto-immune disease, particularly the two commonest forms, Hashimoto and pernicious anaemia. There is no doubt that amongst parents, sibs, and offspring of patients with Hashimoto's disease there are abnormally high numbers with thyroid disease. In 194 relatives of Doniach's series there were 21 cases of typical Hashimoto thyroiditis and 17 of thyrotoxicosis as well as some atypical conditions. Serological tests showed 46 per cent with thyroid antibodies in relatives as against 15 per cent in matched controls, 20 and 8 per cent respectively with gastric antibody, and 10 and 2 per cent with both. Clearly there is some genetic influence on the occurrence of thyroid disease and some common genetic factor that predisposes either to thyroid disease of pernicious anaemia. It is equally striking, however, that in all studies a substantial proportion of unselected individuals ranging from 5 to 15 per cent show thyroid auto-antibodies. Perhaps related to this is the finding that sections of thyroid taken at autopsy from unselected individuals show lymphocytic infiltration in a high proportion of elderly females. It is reasonable to deduce that the thyroid is the most likely target of a local auto-immune response in the body, although only a very small proportion of those in which such a response occurs show any evidence of disease.

Pathogenesis of thyroid disease

No one has provided a satisfactory interpretation of the over-all pattern of thyroid disease and the part played by auto-immunity. Obviously the conditions are complex and to some extent individual to every patient. Further, the possible influence of iodine deficiency and ingestion of goitrogenic natural substances must be kept in mind. Simply because of the absence of any other known etiological factor I shall assume that thyrotoxicosis, Hashimoto's thyroiditis and its end state, myxoedema, are of primary auto-immune origin. The problem, then, is to produce a credible account of pathogenesis that covers the clinical and pathological findings and is not inconsistent with what has emerged from experimental work on animals.

I shall assume, again from the lack of a visible alternative, that thyrotoxicosis results from stimulation by the auto-antibody LATS of hormone receptors normally responding to TSH. The development of Graves's disease has many of the characteristics of an autocatalytic process which may give a clue as to the means of its initiation. The existence of nodular toxic goitre makes it not unreasonable to suggest that in persons genetically predisposed to respond in what may be called auto-immune fashion a local mutation of a thyroid cell to hyperactivity may occur and result in a small nidus of hyperactive descendant cells. All cell surfaces are metabolically active, losing components to the environment and resynthesizing or replacing them from the cytoplasm. A minimal leak of thyroid antigens, including TSH-receptor substance, must be passing normally to local lymph nodes at a level below that needed either to provoke LATS or to induce tolerance sufficient to prevent its production when larger amounts of antigen were available. With the development of a more active source of TSH-receptor molecules, sufficient potential antigen may reach the draining lymph nodes to stimulate antibody production, provided the individual can produce antigen-reactive cells of the right quality. One would guess that right quality meant with the right degree of affinity for the functional groupings of the receptor molecule to produce a stimulus equivalent to that of TSH. The ability to produce such a pattern of combining site could be one genetic quality required to allow hyperthyroidism, but there must be additional requirements.

By hypothesis, once significant amounts of LATS were circulating, thyroid stimulation and hyperplasia would be associated with release of TSH-receptor substance to pass to lymphoid tissue where, acting as an auto-immunogen, it could induce further proliferation of LATS-producing clones. Once significant concentrations of antigen, antibody, and presumably, specific T-immunocytes develop in significant regions of the body, the complex interactions discussed in Chapter 4 will take place. The balance between positive response with proliferation and antibody production on the one hand and negative with inhibition of response (tolerance) on the other will be influenced by these and other factors. By hypothesis, in the auto-immune condition the balance is pushed to the positive side and there will be an autocatalytic quality about the process, whereas in the normal individual an early development of tolerance or negative feedback by antibody could cut the process down before symptoms were produced. This picture of the pathogenesis of exophthalmic goitre is at present pure hypothesis, but it is a hypothesis which could be tested experimentally with only minor developments of techniques currently in use.

Before leaving this topic one should mention the possibility that functional overaction of other endocrine organs might conceivably have a similar origin by the random appearance of an immune pattern with effective resemblance to the effector configuration of a controlling hormone. There are in fact rare hyperplasias, of unknown etiology and non-malignant in character, affecting adrenal cortex, and parathyroid with corresponding symptoms of functional overactivity. Amongst pituitary disorders, acromegaly, some primary cases of Cushing's syndrome and diabetes insipidus might be candidates for consideration. The justification of such an approach is simply that apart from malignant disease the only way by which somatic change in a single cell can initiate disease is for it to involve an immunocyte clone reacting with an organ-specific antigenic determinant.

To pass to the more conventional type of localized auto-immune disease as exemplified in Hashimoto's disease, we can start with the well-known fact that many cases of Graves's disease show lymphocytic infiltration and can sometimes quieten down to give the typical Hashimoto syndrome. Most cases of Hashimoto's disease develop insidiously and approximately 10 per cent of normal people show circulating antibody to one or other thyroid antigen. Again we can assume that a variety of thyroid components are passing in trace amounts to draining lymph nodes. They would include thyroglobulin and the specific cytoplasmic antigen. As in all such situations, the balance between proliferation, tolerance, and inactivity will be a delicately balanced one with any 'genetic tendency to auto-immunity' swinging the balance toward proliferation. This holds for T- and B-systems and in most cases both types of cell are produced with similar specificity. By hypothesis, Hashimoto's disease results from the entry of auto-immune T-immunocytes into the substance of the target organ with much the same sequence of changes as is seen in experimental allergic encephalitis or a tuberculin reaction. Many non-specific monocytes and lymphocytes must take part. The presence of germinal centres (which are very common in Hashimoto thyroids) and plasma cells might suggest that B-type memory cells, tuned to thyroid antigens, find the initiated lesions a suitable site for proliferation. There is also increased activity and numerous germinal centres in the draining lymph nodes of some cases, but there seems to be no positive evidence that the germinal centres in either site contain immunocytes reactive with thyroid antigens.

Since antibodies to both thyroglobulin and cytoplasmic antigen are much commoner than frank thyroid disease, one must assume that they have no damaging function and may actually serve as an effective inhibitor to the recruitment of specific T-immunocytes. Their presence serves merely to indicate a certain tendency to auto-immune reactions and to suggest that there may be some cellular attack on the thyroid as well.

Gastric atrophy and pernicious anaemia

With the development of simple methods of gastric biopsy by Wood and others, it became evident that diffuse changes in the histological structure of the gastric mucosa were very common in hospital patients. They range from mild superficial gastritis, through a spectrum of conditions with variable degrees of lymphocytic infiltration and of loss of the secreting cells, to severe atrophy of all mucosal structures. In general, one can say that there is a progressive degeneration of the gastric mucosa with age, and a similar increase, at a lower level, in the proportion of individuals with antibody against gastric parietal cells (those which secrete hydrochloric acid and 'intrinsic factor'). There is a much higher incidence of such antibody in patients with gastric atrophy than in those with superficial gastritis, and higher still in those whose gastric atrophy is associated with pernicious anaemia.

There is therefore a strong current trend to look on pernicious anaemia as resulting from progressive auto-immune damage to the parietal cells of the stomach with failure of intrinsic factor production. Lymphocytic infiltration of the mucosa is seen in many cases of chronic atrophic gastritis, and though most investigators have been concerned only with the significance of auto-antibodies against intrinsic factor or parietal cells, it is possible that T-auto-immunocytes are primarily responsible for the atrophy.

Intrinsic factor is a glycoprotein secreted by parietal cells into the stomach cavity which, by uniting with vitamin B12 (cyanocobalamin), allows it to be absorbed from the intestine and play an essential role in the production of red cells. Pernicious anaemia is essentially a failure of B12 to reach the sources of red cell production in the bone marrow. It is an interesting weakness of mammalian physiology that although B12 is an essential food element, neither higher plants nor animals can synthesize it. It is wholly a product of micro-organismal synthesis, and most of the human requirements come from the bacteria in the rumen of sheep and cattle via meat, and particularly liver.

It is probably still not adequately proved that pernicious anaemia is basically an auto-immune disease resulting from the development of T- and B-immunocytes reactive with antigenic determinants present in gastric parietal cells and in the glycoprotein molecules of intrinsic factor, but it remains the best working hypothesis. The actual mechanism by which pernicious anaemia develops is still controversial. Antibody of both types may be found in the blood and in the gastric fluids; lymphocytes and plasma cells, some of which, according to Baur *et al.* (1968), can be shown to contain antibodies against parietal cell antigen and against intrinsic factor, may often be seen in the affected gastric wall. There is some evidence that antibody against intrinsic factor may combine with it in the gastric juice in such a fashion as to render it incapable of facilitating the absorption of B12. This, however, does not throw any light on how the antibody came to be produced.

Having regard to the fact that gastric atrophy is nearly universal with age and commoner than the presence of parietal cell antibody, which in its turn is much more frequent than clinically evident pernicious anaemia, and that only 30–40 per cent of pernicious anaemia cases show antibody against intrinsic factor, we can at least construct a consistent hypothesis along the following lines.

The gastric lining is intermittently subjected to severe physical conditions of low pH, constant turbulence, and contact with potentially irritant materials. Mucosal epithelium is constantly being damaged and replaced; hence intracellular material from disintegrating cells is likely to be liberated into the tissue so that small amounts of various potential auto-antigens are almost constantly moving to the draining lymph nodes. In any individual with the basic genetic character endowing immunocytes with increased resistance to inactivation by antigen, any immunocyte modified by mutation to have a little extra resistance and having the appropriate immune pattern for receptor will find a constantly available source of antigenic determinants to stimulate it to proliferation. Active T-cells will be in a position both to be stimulated to proliferate and when they 'home' to the gastric mucosa produce progressive damage. Corresponding B-cells will be stimulated to antibody production, including IgA production and its liberation into the stomach cavity.

Idiopathic Addison's disease

This is now the commonest form of disease causing complete loss of adrenal cortical function. The evidence for its auto-immune character follows the usual pattern. Histologically there is infiltration by lymphocytes and plasma cells with progressive and apparently irreversible loss of functioning adrenal cells, ending in almost complete atrophy of the organs. The disease is regularly bilateral. Antibody reacting specifically with a microsomal antigen in adrenal cortical cells but not in other tissues is observed in about 50 per cent of cases. There is the usual evidence, clinical or serological, of auto-immune processes involving other organs, notably thyroid and parathyroids, but gastritis and parietal cell antibody are also more common than controls.

TABLE 1. Auto-antibodies observed in patients with localized auto-immune disease

	Percentage of positive tests in patients with				
Auto-antibodies	*Addison's disease*	*Hypoparathyroidism*	*Thyroid disease*	*Pernicious anaemia*	*Normal individuals*
Adrenal (F)	50	15	0	0	0
Parathyroid (F)	26	38	12	..	6
Thryoid antibodies	32	+	85–99	50	4–10
Gastric parietal cell (F)	+	+	30	86	8

F = antibody detected by immunofluorescence.

The most interesting feature of the condition is the relatively frequent association with primary hypoparathyroidism. Of 119 cases of idiopathic Addison's disease 15 showed evidence of hypoparathyroidism and 16 one or other of the types of thyroid disease with auto-immune associations. The cross-reactions of antibodies detected by immunofluorescence in Table 1 leave no doubt that idiopathic Addison's disease has the same status as a localized auto-immune disease as any other of the group.

Liver disease with auto-immune characteristics

There are two liver conditions which are associated with infiltration of lymphocytes and plasma cells in the liver substance and with a variety of 'auto-antibodies' none of which, however, appear to be specific for liver antigens. This provides an *a-priori* case for the two diseases, active chronic hepatitis (ACH), and primary biliary cirrhosis (PBC), to be of auto-immune origin or at least to be associated with secondary auto-immune processes. Typical cases of the two diseases are easily differentiated, but the impression from the literature is strong that there is a continuous spectrum of liver disease associated with auto-immune findings. In view of the established role of alcohol, protein deficiency in childhood, and specific viral infection in producing hepatitis, and in the absence of any means of cultivating the hepatitis viruses, there are major difficulties in deciding on any definite etiological diagnosis for most of the cases seen. In particular, it is still quite obscure whether any or most cases of active chronic hepatitis are essentially sequelae of viral hepatitis. The detection of Australia (Au) or hepatitis-associated

(HA) antigen, which is characteristically found in the blood of serum hepatitis patients, in a proportion of ACH patients points in that direction, but the full significance of the Au antigen is still to be determined.

There have been suggestions that persisting tolerated infections may have a special role in providing conditions for the development of auto-immunity, for example, Hotchin's belief that chronic kidney disease in certain strains of mice infected in this fashion with LCM virus is an auto-immune process. Others have ascribed this lesion, however, to the damaging effect of a viral antigen–antibody complex in the circulating blood.

The general clinical picture of active chronic hepatitis is of recurrent febrile attacks, sometimes with jaundice and other evidence of disordered liver function, usually with progressive over-all deterioration, with about half the patients dead in five years. It has a wide age incidence, but the majority of cases are in young women. Primary biliary cirrhosis tends to involve older women, has a more evenly progressive course, and jaundice is a major symptom.

There are cases of ACH which show symptoms of polyarthritis resembling rheumatoid arthritis, or pleurisy, skin rashes, and splenic enlargement, which could suggest SLE. One section of the group was differentiated as lupoid hepatitis on the basis of a positive LE cell reaction, and a proportion may show rheumatoid factor. There is usually an excess of immunoglobulins in the serum. No type of antibody is diagnostic of either ACH or PBC and none of the antibodies recorded are specific for liver. A complement fixation test with cellular extracts from human liver or kidney, the AICF test, is commonly positive but in this test several different antibodies are involved. Probably the dominant one is directed against mitochondrial protein and can also be detected by immunofluorescence. There is the usual finding that such patients show a higher proportion of thyroid and gastric parietal cell antibodies than paired normal controls. Antibody to smooth muscle, shown by immunofluorescence, is relatively common in both liver diseases and rare in other conditions.

One can feel confident that future study of these liver conditions will in some ways provide a bridge between the generalized diseases such as SLE and local auto-immune disease. The first requirement, however, is to develop satisfactory ways to isolate and identify the hepatitis viruses and to measure the corresponding antibodies. A good start has been made with the detection of the Australia antigen, but its significance is proving difficult to define. The interrelationships of chronic infection with immunological anomalies is one of the potentially important areas of medicine that are almost wholly unexplored.

Myasthenia gravis and the thymus

Myasthenia gravis is a neurological disease affecting predominantly young women, characterized by easy fatigue of muscles, with drooping of the eyelids (ptosis), a characteristic sign. The weakness is ascribed to a neuromuscular block and is diagnosed by recognizing the short-lasting recovery of muscular power when a neostigmine derivative, 'Tensilon', is injected intravenously.

By a combination of largely irrelevant circumstances it was discovered that thymectomy often resulted in a significant improvement and that sections of thymus showed a highly characteristic picture of lymphocytic infiltration in the medulla with numerous germinal centres. This was typical of most cases in young women, but in some 20–30 per cent of patients, particularly in men, the thymus was found to be largely replaced by tumour. These thymomas are usually of non-malignant character, sections showing a rather wide range of cell types in various combinations of epithelial cells, spindle cells, and lymphocytes. Not all thymomas are associated with myasthenia gravis, but when they are the disease tends to be severe and serological signs are well marked. Results of removal of thymoma (and associated thymus) were beneficial in some cases, but not so frequently as in the non-thymoma cases. Simpson's survey in abbreviated form is given in Table 2.

The characteristic serological finding in myasthenia gravis is the presence of antibody binding with the I-bands of striated muscle and of the so-called myoid cells of thymic medulla. Antibody in significant amount is found in only 30 per cent of cases and is usually of higher titre when a thymoma is present. Surgical removal of a thymoma has little or no effect on antibody titre. Perhaps an even more significant finding is that, according to Strauss, 12 of 51 thymomas *not* associated with myasthenia gravis showed high titres of myoid antibody. To complete the clinico-pathological picture of myasthenia gravis, lymphocytic infiltration, usually rather trivial, in skeletal muscle and some structural abnormalities of the neuromuscular junction have been noted.

TABLE 2. Results in 494 cases of myasthenia gravis (Simpson) (percentage)

	Thymoma		No thymoma	
	Remission	*Death from myasthenia*	*Remission*	*Death from myasthenia*
Operated	25	58	62	10
Controls	27	63	33	67

In view of Goldstein's experimental work, described below, it is important to emphasize the curious relationship to thyroid disease. There is a frequent association of thyrotoxicosis with myasthenia gravis. In two series of myasthenias 5·3 per cent and 8 per cent had thyrotoxicosis. Hashimoto's disease and hypothyroidism are at least as common and about 25 per cent had thyroid auto-antibodies.

The most serious attempt to provide an experimental model of myasthenia gravis is that of Goldstein and Whittingham, who immunized guinea-pigs with calf thymus extracts in Freund's complete adjuvant. This resulted in an infiltration of the thymic medulla with lymphocytes but no appearance of germinal centres. There was moderate histological damage to muscle but no development of myoid antibody. A proportion (6 out of 24) of immunized animals gave an electromyographic response which showed a significant rise with neostigmine administration. Prior thymectomy in nineteen guinea-pigs subsequently immunized gave none which showed a neostigmine-reversible reduction in myographic response. Largely on the basis of this result, Goldstein postulates a substance, 'thymin', present in normal thymuses and released in abnormal amount from thymuses auto-immunologically damaged. So far this work has not been confirmed. Vetters *et al.* (1970) failed to show any neuromuscular block in such animals.

I find myself sympathetic to Goldstein's attitude that the agent responsible for the myasthenia is a hormone-like agent produced by the thymus and not an auto-antibody. It follows that it is also produced more profusely by those thymomas which are active in this respect, irrespective of whether they are associated with myoid antibody production or not. I am not competent to assess the neurophysiological data presented in Goldstein's and Mackay's monograph on the human thymus, but will provisionally accept the evidence that myasthenia is due to a hormone-like action on the neuromuscular junction, reversible or irreversible, and that the hormone is produced in pathologically altered thymuses.

Accepting provisionally that the effect on the neuromuscular junction is hormonal rather than due to any immunological factor, the main features requiring interpretation are the nature of the antigen toward which the main antibody is directed, the significance of the germinal centres in the thymic medulla and the curious relationship to thymoma. Any interpretation must be speculative and directed more to defining areas for further study than toward any dogmatic explanation.

The auto-antibody reactive with the I band of skeletal muscle and with certain epithelial cells of the thymic medulla is of primary interest in relation to the reactive thymic cells. These are now regarded as myoid cells showing a basic structure similar to skeletal muscle. It is also quite common to see, in mouse thymuses at least, ciliated epithelium of bronchiolar type and sometimes a patch of what appear to be parathyroid cells. This suggests that the thymus may retain and occasionally express some of the various potentialities of the branchial regions from which it is derived.

One could picture, therefore, that newly differentiated immunocytes of appropriate quality might find in the thymus itself an unexpected variety of cells carrying specific tissue antigens including one characteristic of muscular tissue. Under some circumstances this could allow an appropriately 'resistant' immunocyte to be stimulated and initiate a 'forbidden' clone. If B-cells were involved, germinal proliferation and antibody production might take place both in the thymus and in draining lymph nodes. The associated thymitis, to which Goldstein ascribes the production of excess agent blocking neuromuscular junctions, could well serve to increase the amount of accessible myoid cell auto-antigen and confer a self-perpetuating character on the process. On the assumption that the main source of 'myoid' antigen was the thymus itself, a reasonable interpretation of the benefit of thymectomy in early cases uncomplicated by thymoma is at hand.

Significance of thymomas

The part played by thymoma is more interesting and more difficult to interpret. The relevant facts in addition to what has already been said are:

1. That when thymoma is associated with myasthenia its removal

with the rest of the thymus by surgery is often quite unsuccessful, both symptoms and serological findings being unaltered.

2. That about a quarter of the cases of thymoma *without* symptoms of myasthenia show myoid auto-antibody.

3. That thymomas are not infrequently associated with hypogammaglobulinaemia (12 per cent), erythroid hypoplasia (weakness of red cell production) (5 per cent), and Cushing's syndrome, the last being characteristic of an unusual type of small cell carcinoma of the thymus. Any may or may not be associated with myasthenia. There are also on record rare instances of association with a wide range of auto-immune diseases.

4. That on rare occasions removal of a thymoma has been followed by the development of myasthenia.

Most of those who have discussed these phenomena have tried to develop some type of interpretation, none of which has been wholly satisfactory. Goldstein, like most authors, regards the thymomas as primary, stating that 'they appear to induce auto-immunization to the myoid antigen contained in certain of the tumour cells'. I have, however, seen no report that tumour cells themselves reacted with the myoid antibody. My own predilection would be to think of the possibility of a LATS-like action against thymic epithelial cells being responsible for the production of some or most thymomas other than those which are frankly malignant. One might postulate that the auto-antibody was directed against a hypothetical receptor substance mediating the pituitary effect on the thymus, which has been demonstrated by Pierpaoli *et al.* (1969). Just as LATS is usually associated with other types of thyroid auto-antibodies, the 'thymoma-stimulus' might only appear in association with other thymic auto-antibodies. The wide variation of associated clinical phenomena points strongly to the almost random presence in the thymus of cells with antigens (or ADs) cross-reactive with those of other tissues. The important conditions, erythroid hypoplasia and acquired agammaglobulinaemia, both suggest an impact on bone marrow stem cells. Such tumours are more often composed of spindle cells than those responsible for myasthenia, and Goldstein considers that secretion by the tumour of a substance inhibiting maturation of stem cells is the most likely explanation. The obvious alternative is to postulate a cross-reaction of an auto-immune process between a thymic antigen, perhaps the receptor protein stimu-

TABLE 3. Combinations of auto-immune responses in relation to symptoms of myasthenia gravis (MG)

Symptoms of MG	Auto-immune responses *MY*	*EP.PRO*	*ERY*	*AγG*
+	−	−	−	−
+	+	−	−	−
+	+	+	−	−
−	+	+	−	−
−	−	+	+	−
+	+	+	+	−
−	−	+	+	+
−	−	+	−	+

MY = Antibody reactive with muscle and myoid cells.

EP.PRO = Antibody postulated as stimulating thymo-epithelial proliferation with thymoma production.

ERY = Immune response against erythroblasts.

AγG = Acquired agammaglobulinaemia.

lating epithelial proliferation and vital stem-cell antigenic determinants. If one adds to this the likelihood that the development of a tumorous proliferation of thymic epithelial cells will have local effects equivalent to Goldstein's thymitis and in any case will only arise in persons predisposed to auto-immune disease, a broad approach to the problem becomes available. It is implicit on such a view that in this constellation of auto-antibodies and ADs there could be a variety of failures of cross-reaction as well as positive results. An approximate tabulation of the findings recorded in Goldstein's monograph is shown in Table 3. It would hardly be appropriate to try to apply the point of view to all the situations that have been described, but there is one experimental approach which the hypothesis seems to call for.

Just as myoid cells were recognized in the thymus by immunofluorescence, it seems important to determine whether, amongst the numerous and rather nondescript epithelial cells in the human thymus, there are examples reacting with any of the many other organ-specific human auto-antibodies that are now available. A study of pathological thymuses with and without thymoma along such lines could be very valuable.

Other possible local auto-immune diseases

More than one editor interested in the changing pattern of medical science has commented on the influence of fashion in the interpretation of human disease. When a condition seems to have no obvious cause it tends to be placed provisionally in the currently popular pigeon hole. It is probably only a slight exaggeration to say that over the last fifty years such conditions have been ascribed in sequence to 'septic foci', 'psychosomatic processes', 'auto-immunity', and now 'slow viruses'.

Multiple sclerosis can serve as an example which at the moment is moving from auto-immunity to slow virus without any really legitimate reason for the change. The move has been strongly influenced by work on three diseases which have already been discussed in Chapter 6 as the current prototypes of slow virus disease. They are scrapie in sheep; the strange, lethal disease, kuru, that was spread by cannibalism in the New Guinea Highlands; and a rare cosmopolitan disease of the brain associated with premature senile dementia, hemiparesis, and other signs of brain damage (Creutzfeld–Jakob disease).

The pathology of multiple sclerosis is quite different from kuru or Creutzfeld–Jakob disease, but neither has it any close resemblance to experimental auto-immune disease of the central nervous system nor to the human disease (Guillain–Barré syndrome) which has the best credentials as an auto-immune disease. Undoubtedly there will be continuing study of multiple sclerosis, both for evidence of an infectious agent and for signs of auto-immune processes. The elucidation of its etiology will be a landmark in the history of medicine, but at the present time there is no justification for discussing the possibilities in a book concerned only with general aspects of auto-immune disease.

Amongst the possible auto-immune diseases of the nervous system, the acute polyneuritis of the Guillain–Barré syndrome is a disease that comes on without obvious cause and progresses at varying speed. Clinically it shows as an ascending paralysis, starting with the legs. Sometimes in the form known as Landry's paralysis it rapidly gives rise to complete and fatal muscular paralysis. More often the progress comes to a standstill and slow improvement begins, often leading to complete recovery. The lesions are in the peripheral nerves and show leucocytic infiltration, amongst other changes.

Evidence that this is an auto-immune disease is drawn from the finding of raised protein levels in the cerebrospinal fluid, an experimental model in the rabbit produced by injection of nerve tissue and adjuvants and the recent demonstration of reactive lymphocytes in the blood. The last approach, due to Knowles *et al.* (1969), made use of a basic protein extracted from human peripheral nerve tissue which stimulated lymphocytes to commence mitotis when they were obtained from patients with this disease but was inert against cells from normal patients or those with chronic peripheral neuritis of other types.

A brief account may be given of two ophthalmological conditions which may follow surgical or accidental damage to the eye. The so-called phaco-anaphylaxis results from the liberation of lens protein during cataract extraction.

Sympathetic ophthalmia usually follows a penetrating wound of the eye with tissue disorganization and granuloma formation. At times that may vary from a month to several years a similar acute inflammatory condition may arise in the uninjured eye. Early treatment with corticosteroids is usually effective in preventing further development of the 'sympathetic' lesion.

Here the position seems to be simply that lens protein and other special eye proteins are rigidly segregated antigens under normal conditions and behave essentially as foreign proteins when they are liberated into traumatized tissue. It is possible that predisposition toward auto-immune disease would increase the likelihood of such occurrences.

CHAPTER 12

Pathogenesis of auto-immune disease

Everything I have written on immunological topics for the last twenty years or more has been concerned with the need for recognition of the difference between self, i.e. cells, cell products, and macromolecules whose structure and chemical pattern is genetically proper to the body, and not-self. Once the need and capacity to recognize such differences has arisen it is axiomatic that means must also be available to rid the body of the alien material. That is virtually a definition of the scope of immunology. Auto-immune disease and auto-immune aspects of disease—and since there is never a disease that can be ascribed to a unitary cause the two phrases are virtually synonymous—result from some inadequacy or positive malfunction of those mechanisms for recognition and disposal.

In this chapter I have tried to bring together the general concepts of the forbidden clone approach, many of which have been introduced and elaborated in relation to some specific aspects in earlier chapters. The first requirement is to recapitulate teaching on the normal mechanisms of intrinsic tolerance as discussed in Chapter 4 and the various possibilities by which one or more of these can be overcome, giving opportunity for potential or overt disease.

If the modern approach to immunological theory is accepted, there must inevitably be immune patterns produced which can react with some of the countless potential antigens present in the body. Any mechanism by which specific immune patterns are produced which can react with unknown, i.e. unexperienced, antigenic determinants (ADs) must necessarily be of the general nature of a random diversification of patterns. This must automatically generate many patterns reactive with potential antigenic determinants in the body.

All the work that has been done on intrinsic tolerance as manifested in mice derived from blastocyst chimeras or on experimentally induced perinatal tolerance shows conclusively that removal of the capacity to do immunological damage is not a direct genetic process but one which goes on actively during embryonic and later development and is adjusted to requirements. The very fact that such production of chimeras is possible shows how flexible and adaptive the machinery must be. It is to be expected that no single process will be adequate, and for some years I have used the phrase 'a fail-safe system' to convey the need for back-up controls if some primary mechanism fails. An excellent example of the complexities of tolerance and the part secondary fail-safe factors can play is to be found in a recent paper from the Hellströms' laboratory. They used allophenic mice in which strains *A* (C3H) and *B* (C57Bl) were fused, as a source of lymph node cells, and showed that these allophenic cells had significantly higher cytotoxic effect against parental cells *A* or *B* than had lymph node cells from F1 *A*/*B*s or the opposite parent. The excess cytotoxicity which was not of a very high order could be neutralized with allophenic serum. The conclusion seems justified that 'a concomitant immunity and serum blocking effect rather than a central failure of the immune response may mediate some aspects of tolerance'.

To recapitulate some of what has been discussed earlier, with a more direct attention to immunopathology, natural tolerance, experimental chimeric tolerance, and auto-immune disease are all primarily concerned with ADs carried by body cells, and immunological damage to cells is predominantly mediated by T-immunocytes. We must first, then, look at the ways in which T-cell activity is manifested and how its activity can be prevented. For the time being we can think of T-immunocytes as a legitimate single category, all the members being derived from the descendants of stem cells which were differentiated in the thymus. As a reasonable working assumption, most forms of local auto-immune disease result from the presence in the body of adequately large clone(s) with immune receptors which have a relatively high affinity for one or more ADs of the target cells. It is accepted that in the normal individual there are no such clones, although T-immunocytes must occasionally emerge with an immune pattern reactive with the same ADs. Such cells fail to initiate clonal proliferation on contact with AD for one or other of the reasons previously discussed, viz. destruction, sterile activation, or functional inhibition.

The immunocyte, when first differentiated, has the form of a cortical thymocyte necessarily possessing the full range of surface components characteristic of such cells, many of which are potentially antigenic. Whatever the means by which the receptor substance is synthesized and delivered to the surface, if in the process it encounters and combines with cell material, then the cell cannot become an immunocyte. It is immaterial whether it dies forthwith or passes to the circulation where it will necessarily be unresponsive to any type of specific stimulation. When there is no obstruction of this sort, the receptors develop on the surface to bring a newly differentiated immunocyte into existence. The cell will still have to be tested against any other potential AD produced by cells in its immediate environment or elsewhere.

It is a likely assumption that only in certain physiological states of the cell is it susceptible to *lethal* contact with its specific AD and there is in fact evidence that death of lymphocytes in thymus and germinal centres takes place predominantly in the immediately post-mitotic phase. The simplest deduction is that if effective contact is made when the cell is at a certain stage of its mitotic cycle, in the S premitotic phase, contact is usually lethal, while if the cell is in the resting condition the same stimulus may have other effects.

A variety of rules no doubt exist by which the results of receptor AD contact are modified by the affinity of union, the proportion of receptors occupied, and by the time sequence in relation to mitosis at which receptors are stimulated. It is easy enough to use such parameters to work out conditions which would account for something equivalent to low zone and high zone tolerance in the B system, but there is simply no direct experimental material.

The basic hypothesis of the origin of auto-immune disease would then become as follows:

It depends on the emergence of a clone or a small number of clones of T-immunocytes capable of damaging interaction with normal cells of the organ or tissue involved. Each clone is initiated from a cell which (*a*) has developed an immune receptor adequately reactive with an accessible component of the organ or cell type involved, and (*b*) as a result of somatic mutation or of a sequence of germinal and somatic mutations the newly differentiated immunocyte is anomalously resistant to inactivation by AD contact. Under conditions which would ensure that a normal immunocyte of this reactivity would be eliminated, the mutant cell will proliferate to produce a forbidden clone. As in every immunological context, the difference will never be absolute; it is a difference in the balance of probabilities as between proliferation and elimination.

Many investigations have given evidence of genetic factors being involved in auto-immune disease and I have found it useful for many

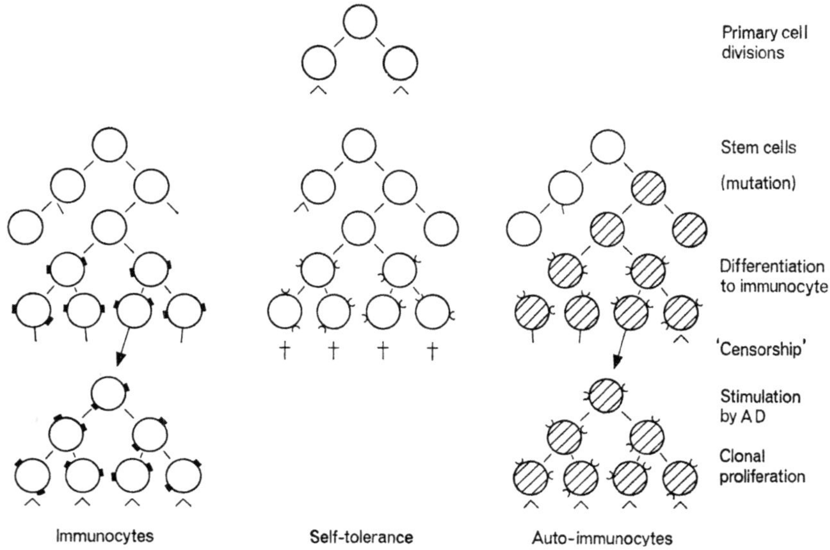

FIG. 21. Simplified diagram to suggest the processes by which clones of immunocytes develop or fail to develop. Two types of receptor are shown emerging with differentiation to immunocyte.
Black rectangle = specific for some foreign AD. Two-pronged = specific for an accessible potential AD in the body. Shading indicates the result of increased resistance to the 'censorship' by which tolerance is established.

purposes to think of auto-immune disease as resulting whenever a certain sequence of mutant genes develops in an immunocyte of the right immune pattern. It is immaterial whether the mutational event is a germinal one that may have occurred a thousand years before and at what stages of development the somatic mutations take place. Burch has suggested that the number of anomalous genes needed may vary considerably from one human auto-immune disease to another, but for simplicity we may assume that three, *a*, *b*, and *c*, are needed. As in all relatively unsophisticated genetic discussions, *a* covers any mutant gene which has an equivalent functional effect, and similarly for *b* and *c*. It is also necessary, of course, that the immunocyte on differentiation carry an immune pattern corresponding to a significant 'self' antigenic determinant. Since this is functionally equivalent to a somatic mutation, we add *s* as an additional requirement for the emergence of a forbidden pathogenic clone.

This discussion of a T-immunocyte could in principle be applied similarly to a B-cell. It will be complicated, however, by the special interaction of B- and T-immunocytes necessary for the production by

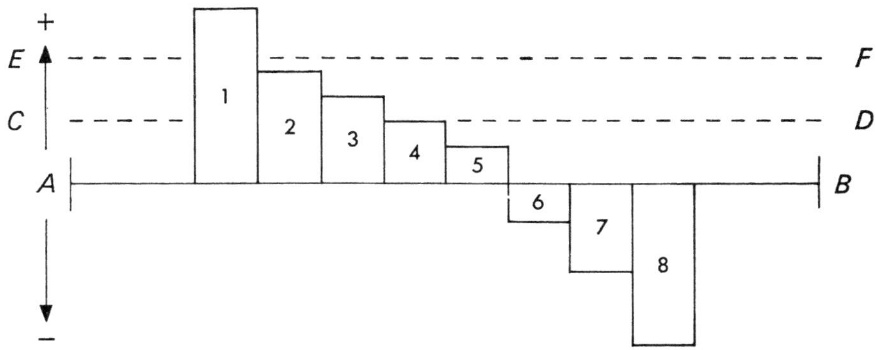

FIG. 22. A schema to illustrate the effect of random mutation on the 'point of balance' between immune response + and tolerance —. See text.

the B-cells of certain types of antibody. I believe that in the absence of knowledge about T- and B-cell interaction in auto-immune conditions nothing will be lost if we make the assumption that forbidden clones of B-cells arise in precisely the same fashion except that differentiation of the (*a*, *b*, *c*, *s*) stem cell to a T-immunocyte takes place in the thymic cortex, to a B-immunocyte 'somewhere else'. It will follow that if the sequence of mutation is completed early in embryonic life there may be a substantial number of (*a*, *b*, *c*, *s*) stem cells differentiating into equivalent T- and B-cells. Any requirements for co-operation could therefore be fulfilled. It is also possible that the final mutation *c* might not occur until immediately before or even after differentiation.

An alternative approach more readily expressed in simple line diagrams may assist in clarifying the intrinsically rather difficult concepts of the forbidden clone and the interaction of genetic and somatic genetic changes. This is to simplify the position to the limit and confine attention to the two significant results of first contact of immunocyte with its corresponding AD. Either the cell reacts positively, giving rise to a descendant clone, or negatively, by physical or functional elimination. It is clear from the facts that which alternative is chosen depends on many parameters relative to the physiological condition of the cell, the mode of presentation of AD and the local micro-environment. If we standardize all but one of the parameters concerned, then we can let a line *AB* represent the level of the remaining parameter corresponding to the balance point between + and − reactions (Fig. 22).

If one accepts the possibility that a variety of somatic mutational changes will incidentally change the neutral point for the cell in one direction or another, this can be represented on the figure by moving *AB* correspondingly. The changed levels are shown for 8 hypothetical mutants. Nos. 6, 7, 8, being on the – side, will be destroyed by antigenic contact, but 1, 2, 3, 4, 5 will be more liable to proliferate. At some level, *EF*, the resistance to destruction will be such that the immunocyte concerned can be positively stimulated by a 'self' antigenic determinant and give rise to a forbidden clone.

It is a simple extension that if a germ line mutation in a certain animal affected *all* immunocytes to an extent equivalent to the somatic mutant 4, so raising *AB* to *CD*, two further grades of mutant could initiate forbidden clones. Similar reasoning could be applied to variation in regard to any other relevant parameter. In other words, the number of forbidden clones that can emerge will increase with each base-line change in the genetic character toward resistance against inactivation by antigen.

Auto-immune haemolytic anaemia

Emergence of the initiating cells, which we can call T- or B-auto-immunocytes, and their capacity to pass the initial censorship process is only the first stage. Obviously no symptoms, not even any auto-antibody production, will be possible until the forbidden clones have been enlarged to some threshold level. That process will have its own requirements, depending largely on the accessibility of the target cell AD or, in the instances where auto-antibodies play a symptom-producing role, the special qualities of the auto-antigen. Of the possible target cells the circulating red cell is much the most accessible and auto-immune haemolytic anaemia can be the first example for discussion. It has the additional virtues that a laboratory model exists in the NZB mouse and there is a phenocopy, as it were, in the positive Coombs test of patients on α-methyldopa and a similar condition associated with infection by *Mycoplasma pneumoniae*.

The spleen is the principal graveyard of red cells and for this and many other reasons we can concentrate on what happens in the spleen in the auto-immune anaemias. It is still by no means clear how the effete red cell is recognized, removed, and disintegrated in the spleen. In all probability there is a surface change associated with ageing which facilitates phagocytosis of the red cell by splenic macrophages. Neither is much known directly about how the haemagglutinins and haemolysins are produced when foreign red cells are administered intravenously. By analogy with other situations, one assumes that in the course of disintegration of the foreign cells in splenic macrophages many types of antigenic fragments are made available for contact with immunocytes of appropriate type amongst the lymphocytic population. Depending on the several factors mentioned earlier, the antigen reactive cells will be either stimulated to proliferate or rendered specifically non-reactive by physical destruction or in some other way. In general, the larger the bulk of red cells, the more likely will be the destruction or conversion to tolerance of a proportion of reactive immunocytes.

In this connection it is appropriate to refer again to the unique character of NZB mice in their response to sheep red cells. Unlike other mouse strains, the response, i.e. number of plaque-forming cells (PFC), rose as a function of antigen dose to the largest practical amount (10^9 cells) instead of showing an optimal dose at 10^7–10^8. Fitting into the same general pattern is the failure of NZB mice to be rendered tolerant by injections of particle-free foreign gammaglobulins. Here at least we have a clear hint that there is a genetic characteristic which involves all antigen-reactive cells of NZB which renders them more resistant than normal to being 'turned off' by excess antigen. We could well regard this quality as the *a* of our genetic formulation.

Clearly, however, neither in NZB mice nor in human patients with auto-immune haemolytic anaemia (AHA) is the disease a straightforward genetic characteristic. Additional somatic changes are needed to give rise to an initiating cell with both the appropriate immune receptor and a much increased resistance to inactivation by the normal tolerance-producing processes. Once such a cell appears there will be a greatly increased likelihood of the emergence of a frankly pathogenic clone. If the suggestion stands up that there is a specially vulnerable period at one phase of the mitotic cycle while at other phases stimulation favours proliferation, a highly complex set of stochastic equations involving parameters not yet capable of quantitation would be needed to express the probability of emergence into disease. The practical implication is that it becomes highly probable that at some stage of the process only a single clone of auto-antibody-producing cells will be present in significant amount. With appropriate serological study of the Coombs antibody, this can be established both in human and in murine disease.

The frequent production of a typical direct Coombs reaction in persons taking regular doses of α-methyldopa suggests that the presence of this drug or a stage in its metabolic disposal can influence the result of antigen-immune receptor contact in increasing resistance to destruction, in other words it has a basically similar action to the gene *c*. One would presume that an adequate concentration of the drug must be present in the micro-environment in the spleen where contacts take place. It must be remembered, however, that the production of a Coombs test is not equivalent to AHA either in patients on the drug or in the rare instances where a positive test is found in persons who appear otherwise to be in perfect health. It is, however, a step on the way. Amongst the rather small numbers of patients developing AHA in England in the 1965–6 period a quite disproportionate number of them were being treated with α-methyldopa. It was suggested that about 0·02 per cent of patients treated with the drug developed AHA. Here another genetic or somatic genetic factor must be involved. The nature of the phenotypic process by which a rather regular production of a Coombs reaction, i.e. of auto-antibody without haemolytic anaemia, is converted into clinical disease remains to be established.

Until benign Coombs positive conditions were recognized, the usual intepretation of AHA was that it was *due to* the auto-antibody which, acting as an opsonin, caused accelerated destruction of red cells before the end of their normal physiological life. This cannot be the whole story, though it is certainly possible that some types of high affinity antibody once bound to the circulating red cells would ensure their rapid removal and breakdown in the spleen. The most likely interpretation of the difference between the benign condition with a positive Coombs test and the clinically evident AHA is that any immunocyte, either T or B, with an immune receptor of an affinity which would make its descendant clone pathogenic will be correspondingly more prone to destruction by contact when in the potentially vulnerable phase. Relatively low affinity antibody will be characteristic of the benign condition. Only when a rare additional somatic mutation (which can be taken as equivalent to *b*) eventuates will a 'high affinity' immunocyte survive contact with antigen and be in a position to give rise to a clone-producing pathogenic antibody.

Another feature of AHA which may be relevant is its age incidence, more particularly the fact that alone amongst well-defined auto-immune diseases it can involve infants. That it should do so suggests, first, that always one, and perhaps two, of the necessary mutant genes must be inherited or produced very early in the stem cell line so that many candidates for final activation are present soon after birth. The other feature worth mentioning is that for reasons that need not be elaborated three such infants resistant to all standard treatment were subjected to thymectomy and made a rapid recovery. In one the thymus contained numerous plasmablasts actively multiplying. In the other two the thymus was shrunken, inactive, and histologically uninformative. Recovery after thymectomy *may* have been completely coincidental, but 3 out of 3 successes suggests that this is unlikely. Hypotheses could be elaborated, but in the absence of any way to detect immunocytes of auto-immune clones they would have to remain sterile. To a certain extent this holds also for *any* discussion of AHA from the forbidden clone point of view. Nevertheless, the approach involving a sequence of germinal and/or somatic mutations (*a*, *b*, *c*, *s*) fits a wide sequence of phenomena in a fashion which seems likely to be better than any alternative set of suggestions.

A related topic worth brief discussion concerns the cold agglutinins found in *Mycoplasma pneumoniae* infections ('atypical pneumonia'). These have recently been authoritatively ascribed to the fact that the particular red cell antigenic determinant *I* corresponds to the blood group specificity I, characteristic of all but a very small proportion of human red cells after the neonatal stage is passed. The AD *I* cross-reacts with ADs present on *Mycoplasma pneumoniae*, streptococcus MG, and *Listeria monocytogenes*, and we must regard the cold agglutinin as arising essentially by the stimulation of immunocytes of the appropriate class by the extrinsic antigen. As in the case of the harmless Coombs reaction, it appears that when an antibody reactive with but quite innocuous toward a body cell is involved, tolerance being in a sense unnecessary, there is no destructive contact between AD and ARC. Equally, just as in the α-methyldopa situation, an occasional case of haemolytic anaemia develops in mycoplasma infections. When this occurs the highly reversible coating of cold agglutinin at body temperature on the red cell acts to allow an otherwise inadequate set of conditions, arising one assumes by a somatic mutational process involving immunocytes, to develop full haemolytic anaemia. It conforms entirely to the hypothesis that such haemolytic anaemias are short-lasting and cure themselves spontaneously as the infection is overcome.

Perhaps one further example should be added: the haemolytic

anaemia is induced in a small proportion of patients receiving the drug stibophen. Analysis *in vitro* indicates that a high affinity antibody specific for the drug is present in the patient's serum. It has no action on red cells in the absence of stibophen in the system. The process in the test-tube system comprising stibophen, patient's antibody, normal human red cells, and complement probably provides a legitimate model of what takes place in the body. The first step is that stibophen, perhaps held loosely on some protein carrier, combines firmly with antibody. The complex is then adsorbed to the red cell surface, attracts complement components, and the red cell haemolyses. Since no AD natural to the red cell is concerned, the process has no direct relevance to AHA. The rarity of the condition does suggest, however, that only a rare immune pattern capable of avid union with the drug hapten but not susceptible to any tolerigenic effect is capable of initiating an effective clone. In a sense such a cell could be more or less equivalent to the initiatory immunocyte founding an auto-immune clone except that the pattern is not a self one.

Auto-immune disease involving a specific organ

The only other condition which need be elaborated here at any length is the general one of auto-immune disease directed against a specific target organ. Thyroid and adrenals would be the obvious prototypes, but with appropriate regard for special features the approach would be broadly similar to auto-immune processes in any local organ. It would be convenient to limit discussion to auto-immune disease confined to a single localized organ, but it is characteristically rare to find auto-immune disease in one organ without some evidence of involvement of other organs.

In local auto-immune disease diagnosis is normally based on a combination of evidence of functional inadequacy of the affected organ plus the presence of auto-antibodies relevant to the organ. In the course of such work it has become very clear that if one uses a standard battery of tests for auto-antibody, certain general patterns will emerge after a few hundred persons, normal or in hospital for an average spectrum of complaints, are tested. They can be tabulated as follows:

1. A proportion of normal individuals will give low titre positive reactions with the common tissue-specific antigens from thyroid and gastric parietal cells respectively. Antinuclear factor (ANF) will also be found in a proportion.

2. The percentage of nominally healthy patients showing one or more of these positive tests increases almost linearly with age.

3. When there is well-established evidence of functional defect in an organ compatible with auto-immune disease, it is common to find ±80 per cent of such patients showing the corresponding type of tissue-specific auto-antibody and a considerably greater percentage with other positive tests than in comparable normal people.

As has been discussed earlier (p. 163), auto-antibodies are commonly found, but there is little or nothing to suggest that they play more than a minor role in pathogenesis. The affected organs are characteristically infiltrated with lymphocytes, plasma cells, and other mononuclear cells. I am not aware of specific examinations for mast cells (which are not recognizable in routine haematoxylin-eosin sections) except in ulcerative colitis, where they are numerous. In heavy infiltrations, particularly in the thyroid, it is common to find germinal centres, but I know of no investigations to determine whether the *a-priori* thought that each represents a proliferating clone of B-immunocytes specific for a tissue antigen has any validity. By analogy with delayed hypersensitivity, the infiltration should correspond to a small proportion of specific T-immunocytes associated with a majority of non-specific 'bystanders and fellow travellers', but again direct experiment in man is impossible.

Any attempt to construct a plausible account of pathogenesis will depend almost wholly on analogy with conditions in AHA and with what is observed in the animal models in which disease is produced either by injection of various tissue extracts or purified components in FCA, or by induction of graft versus host reactions, usually by the 'parent into F1' technique. Since none of these three conditions chosen for analogy are closely related to human local auto-immune disease or to each other, our speculative outline of pathogenesis is offered only because no better interpretation has yet been possible.

The determinants of local auto-immune disease on our general approach would be, first, the emergence of immunocytes of appropriate character and, second, the development of a source of specific antigens to stimulate their proliferation. The essential difference from the AHA situation is the initial presumption that most of the ADs in question are inaccessible, i.e. they are not normally available in sufficient amount to act either as tolerigenic or immunogenic stimuli. Looking at the situation teleologically, one can in addition feel certain that under normal chances of life, trauma or infection will upset local equilibria sufficiently to release significant amounts of tissue-specific ADs on some occasions. It would seem a necessity for survival that this should not induce a progressive specific immunological infiltration of the organ so damaged. Again some form of fail-safe control must be incorporated to maintain normality. It might be of the type envisaged by Hellström, where any proliferative stimulus to T-cells is countered by concomitantly produced blocking antibody. Whatever the mechanism, it seems likely that for it to be ineffective would require some extra quality of resistance to control in the T-immunocyte concerned. In other words, a generally similar situation must obtain as holds when the auto-antigen is fully accessible.

As before, the critical position is the balance between stimulation to proliferation or to tolerance (including destruction) and the basic hypothesis that this may be pushed in one direction or the other by relatively minor mutations in the cell line (germinal and/or somatic, and probably of many different kinds) and also by changes in the relevant micro-environments. Following the general rule, no somatic mutation is significant unless it results in proliferation of the mutant form. Anything that fosters tolerance, i.e. non-proliferation or death, will mean that the affected cells vanish at a greater rate than normal. Any abnormality in the opposite direction, with increased vigour of proliferation and resistance to destruction by large amounts of antigen, will favour survival of the line.

The intrinsic quality of the immunocyte, as modified by germ line or somatic genetic processes, is clearly important, but the other factor, the presence of accessible auto-antigen in effective concentration, is equally necessary. This point has been discussed at some length in relation to auto-immune haemolytic anaemia in man and in NZB mice. There the spleen is central as a physiological disposal site for red cells. In localized tissues damaged or effete cells are quietly removed, presumably by phagocytosis, and there will rarely be any significant amounts of free tissue-specific antigens available.

A situation with some analogy to the red cell–spleen system could arise when a nidus of auto-immune damage in the target organ is once established. Once the key assumption is made that auto-immune immunocytes are not subject to inhibition or destruction by high concentrations of the corresponding antigenic determinant, it is easy to visualize an autocatalytic process being initiated. Cytotoxic damage to specific tissue cells would liberate more antigen which, passing to draining lymph nodes, would be in a position to induce proliferation of memory cells of the pathogenic clone. The other possibility, suggested by several authors in regard to homograft immunity, is that any lymphocyte of the clone passing through the inflamed region would be stimulated by antigen and, either locally or in some draining lymph node, produce a descendant population.

It will be obvious that if, say, ten mutant immunocytes capable of initiating localized auto-immune disease of the adrenal are present and randomly distributed amongst the whole lymphoid cell population, the chance of any one of them being trapped in an adrenal capillary and initiating a cytotoxic process will be vanishingly small. It will be equally unlikely that any of the cells should be specifically stimulated by adrenal antigen contacted in lymphoid tissue. But once a small necrotic inflammatory focus is established, there will be a much more significant probability of both occurrences. Obviously, as immunocytes of the line proliferate, there will be a progressive intensification of damage to the organ.

Another implication of this model is that, once a cytotoxic process is initiated, any other potential auto-antigens present in the cells will become accessible to any appropriate immunocytes of either T or B systems. It is very common, for instance, to find at least two types of thyroid auto-antibody in thyrotoxicosis or Hashimoto's disease.

It will be recognized that this approach almost necessarily implies that at least in those genetically predisposed to auto-immune disease there will probably always be occasional immunocytes somewhere in the body which are potentially reactive with one or more of the thousands of potential antigenic determinants in the cells and tissues of the body. Normally they will live out their span without finding the necessary stimulation that could set them to building up a pathogenic or antibody-producing clone. But the situation can change immediately once circumstances provide an abnormal abundance of auto-antigen.

Perhaps the best interpretation of the multiple antibodies of SLE can be sought along similar lines. Anyone who is a potential candidate for SLE would have immunocytes relatively resistant to destruction by antigenic contact and liable to be rendered more so by minor somatic mutation. In the stage preceding any manifestation of disease one can reasonably picture many isolated cells with auto-immune potentialities but in insufficient number to have a chance for any to meet the corresponding AD under appropriate conditions. Possibly by some triggering impact, possibly by the eventual initiating contact of AD and immunocyte where conditions were right, one pictures the initial process taking place in lymphoid tissue. Pathogenic immunocytes, reactive against thymic cortex and perhaps any other region of lymphocyte proliferation, would in the course of that activity produce a progressively increasing concentration of fragments with potential ADs. For a time at least this could allow any potential initiator of a pathogenic clone a greater opportunity to be stimulated by the appropriate AD.

Ectopic production of antigens by tumours

A set of phenomena which seem to be of special importance in understanding the pathogenesis of local auto-immune disease concerns the so-called ectopic production of proteins, hormones, or antigens by some tumours. This has been discussed extensively in a previous book (Burnet, 1970), but some of the aspects relevant to auto-immunity should also be mentioned here.

Any somatic cell carries potentially all the genetic information present in any other cell in the body. Appropriate derepression in principle could allow a skin epithelial cell to produce a pituitary hormone or an immunoglobulin. It is now clear that many tumours, perhaps especially bronchial carcinomas, do in fact produce proteins that are inappropriate for production by bronchial epithelium. If a highly active hormone is produced its effect will be directly evident and most of the reports have dealt with such occurrences. There is, however, no visible reason why hormones should be preferentially produced. Probably any ectopic protein is as likely to be produced and liberated as any other; the difficulty is to recognize the fact. In general, proteins produced will be non-antigenic, but an important exception could be any normally inaccessible tissue-specific protein such as those which provide antigenic determinants concerned in auto-immune diseases. A number of types of organ disease with auto-immune character have been described as being clearly associated with cancer and not due to localized metastases. Dermatomyositis and a variety of neuromyopathies are those most consistently observed, but in addition there are occasional dramatic individual cases. One reported by Litwin and Kunkel concerned a woman with severe rheumatoid arthritis and with very well-developed serological reactions. Routine clinical study showed a typical bronchial carcinoma. This was removed surgically, with rapid disappearance of all symptoms of arthritis and of positive serological tests. Within a year, however, local regrowth of the tumour had occurred and concomitantly the symptoms and auto-antibodies of rheumatoid arthritis returned.

Such occurrences are too rare for any sort of stochastic analysis, but, having regard to the relatively short life history of malignant tumours and the necessarily very small proportion which could be expected to produce any specific protein ectopically, it is a reasonable deduction that genetic abnormality (at the germinal level) is not directly concerned in the process. One must, however, qualify this in regard to the rheumatoid arthritis case. According to Burch, a very large proportion of elderly women show some clinical evidence of rheumatoid arthritis and most may well have in circulation a proportion of cells which in the absence of control could undergo pathogenic proliferation. If the appropriate auto-antigen in rheumatoid arthritis is semi-denatured immunoglobulin in the form of an antigen–antibody complex, it is impossible to guess at the actual nature of the ectopic material produced by the tumour. A close study of proteins actually in the surgically removed specimen might have given the answer.

A somewhat similar case reported by Kahn *et al.* (1966) was of SLE associated with an ovarian dysgerminoma. With removal of the tumour, symptoms of SLE and the serological signs disappeared. The process here is even more difficult to guess.

The part played by antigen–antibody complexes

In any animal living in a normal environment there must be frequent entrance of bacteria and bacterial products into regions of minor trauma and with reasonable certainty occasional leakage of potentially antigenic proteins or polypeptides from the gut. In the process of dealing with these, denatured immunoglobulins in the form of antigen–antibody complexes must develop and one of the standard tolerance requirements is that no reactivity to such denatured immunoglobulins should develop. In a variety of pathological conditions more massive amounts of Ag–Ab complexes will develop, particularly if auto-antibodies against a soluble plasma component are concerned. It is worth looking, therefore, at the fate of antigen–antibody complexes in the body in so far as they may be relevant to the phenomena of auto-immune disease.

Perhaps the simplest instance is the condition that arises in subacute bacterial endocarditis where large numbers of streptococci are growing in 'vegetations' on a previously damaged heart valve. Antibodies against streptococci develop and in due course almost any organism dislodged into the circulation will be coated with antibody immunoglobulin. In most such patients rheumatoid factor, i.e. anti-immunoglobulin, develops but there is no evidence of rheumatoid arthritis, and if the valvular infection is effectively dealt with the rheumatoid factor rapidly disappears. The possibility that bacterial infections, for example, tonsillo-pharyngitis, could provide a stimulus via antibody-coated organisms to the rheumatoid process would revive the old septic focus hypothesis in a new form.

In all serologically positive cases of rheumatoid arthritis there are immunoglobulin–immunoglobulin complexes, usually IgM–IgG. It is orthodox to ascribe much of the pathogenesis to these complexes which have a capacity to produce vasculitis and, either secondary to this or directly, lodge in relation to joint synovia. In most rheumatoid joints leucocytes in synovial fluid contain large and numerous immunoglobulin inclusions. Glomerulonephritis is not, however, a standard complication of rheumatoid arthritis and the circulating complexes do not accumulate at the glomerular basement membrane in the fashion characteristic of SLE.

In SLE and in NZB/W mouse disease the evidence is consistent with most of the damage in the kidney being due primarily to the lodgement of Ag–Ab complexes in which nucleic acids are the important antigens. Complement components presumably play a major part and fibrinogen with fibrin deposition and serum albumin may also accumulate at the same sites.

One could probably summarize the situation by saying that under normal circumstances Ag–Ab complexes are rapidly removed from the body fluids by macrophages where they are mainly broken down and their components returned to the metabolic pool. A small part of the antigen will often play a role in immunological processes. Damage arises when excessive amounts develop and when much of the complexed material remains in the circulation for unduly long periods. Experimental work suggests that Ag–Ab complex, solubilized in excess of antigen, is the most potent agent of kidney damage, but it is not easy to identify such a situation in SLE.

Conclusion

After nearly fifteen years' almost uninterrupted thought about the nature of auto-immune disease I am still convinced that it must be looked at as basically the result of genetic anomaly in lymphoid cells of the immune system. The genetic anomalies may be of germinal origin in part, but always include one or more of somatic mutational origin, and if an auto-immune cell line is to develop, an appropriate immune pattern must have been generated in the line. The appearance of an initiating cell from which a pathogenic forbidden clone can develop is thus a wholly random occurrence which can be discussed quantitatively only by using stochastic methods such as those of Burch.

The genetic anomalies concern factors still hardly at all understood which determine how contact with a reactive AD stimulates a given immunocyte. Clearly there is a set of alternatives that can be usefully stated as a balance between proliferation to an immunologically active clone and functional elimination leading to tolerance or paralysis. This is undoubtedly over-simplified but nothing seems to be gained by trying to elaborate detail without an experimental basis. The concept of a balance between two alternatives that can be tipped one way or another by a variety of mutational changes in the cell or of physico-chemical changes in the micro-environment is one which can be easily particularized with the emergence of definable parameters and at the same time provides a convenient logical structure against which to co-ordinate empirical findings.

Just as in the closely analogous field of malignant disease, the basic genetic and somatic genetic processes take place in organisms subject to infection and other impacts of the environment and their results are liable to be modified correspondingly. I can see nothing that seriously suggests that any laterally spread virus plays the slightest role in auto-immune disease. If Huebner's concept of an inherent instability in the mammalian genome (as a result of which very rare stochastic episodes result in the construction and release of viral-type structures which may or may not be associated with malignant change) is established for cancer, something similar may emerge in regard to auto-immune disease. I believe, however, that Huebner would agree that, operationally, the concept cannot be differentiated from that of the forbidden clone hypothesis.

As has been emphasized, the emergence of a cell which in principle could initiate a pathogenic clone of immunocytes will only do so if it finds appropriate auto-antigen to stimulate it. In an otherwise normal individual this may be an extremely rare occurrence and there is much to suggest that until an abnormally accessible source of auto-antigen becomes available the auto-immune condition will not develop.

When we move from the initiation of an anomalous clone of immunocytes to the processes by which it produces disease, the influence of the environment will be of varying importance. One should bear in mind that *any* antibody or any clone of T-immunocytes represents the outcome of a stochastic process, and that it is well recognized that the symptoms of many infections are largely determined by immune responses. The behaviour of auto-immune conditions falls into perspective if one arranges a series of diseases that are immunologically mediated in a sequence starting with those in which the immunological effect is almost wholly determined by the environmental impact and ending with a disease like SLE, where the causation is wholly intrinsic. The following sequence should be enough to illustrate the concept.

1. The rash in measles and rubella.
2. Serum sickness.
3. Rheumatic fever and acute glomerulonephritis.
4. Drug purpuras and haemolytic anaemias.
5. Late syphilis, chronic active hepatitis, ?scrapie and kuru.
6. Rheumatoid arthritis.
7. Local auto-immune disease of thyroid or adrenal.
8. Auto-immune haemolytic anaemia.
9. Systemic lupus erythematosus.

CHAPTER 13

Potentialities and limitations of therapy

The diseases that I have included as auto-immune comprise a large and important section of the patients seen in any hospital physician's wards. Methods of preventing and curing such conditions would obviously be of the greatest practical importance. Unfortunately the prospect of success seems at the present to be very limited indeed.

Prevention, in particular, is an almost hopeless task, even in principle, unless future developments indicate that there are more important environmental 'triggers' than we realize. At present there is no approach to diminishing the likelihood of somatic mutation apart from eliminating an infection like syphilis and using cytotoxic drugs with the greatest possible discretion. One of the important terminal aspects of chronic lympho-proliferative disease, the development of auto-immune haemolytic anaemia or thrombocytopenic purpura, appears to be rather frequently a result of therapy for the primary disease with X-irradiation and cytotoxic drugs. Both are known to be potential mutagens and these effects presumably result from the induction of somatic mutations in the exposed cells. This may apply either to the abnormal lymphocytes of the primary disease or to the residual initially normal population.

There may be something to be done in diminishing the incidence or delaying the onset of rheumatoid arthritis by good medical care of general and local infections in childhood and throughout life. Most physicians assume a large part of the syndrome results from the pathogenic action of immunocytes and/or antibodies reacting with partially denatured immunoglobulin. The commonest source of this auto-antigen must be that produced in the course of latent, minor, or acute infections, and even more so when chronic bacterial infection persists anywhere in the body. To deal with such matters is, of course, the recognized function of modern preventive and curative medicine. I should expect that an adequate statistical analysis would show that our success in dealing with infection since, say, 1945 is already showing a reduction in rheumatoid arthritis, but I have found no recorded information on the matter.

Still on the topic of ways by which the accessibility of auto-antigens could be reduced, we might consider the possibility that active chronic hepatitis might be reduced in incidence if environmental sanitation and better injection techniques could sufficiently reduce the frequency of infectious and serum hepatitis.

For the treatment of established disease, the possible approaches that have been considered and tried can be summarized under four headings:

1. The use of cytotoxic drugs designed to destroy any rapidly proliferating clones of cells.

2. The inhibition of the stimulus arising from contact of cell receptor with AD, by corticosteroids.

3. The use of drugs to counter the liberation or the damaging action of pharmacologically active substances from responding immunocytes or cells secondarily involved.

4. The elimination, if it is surgically practical, of any source providing an excessive amount of the auto-antigen.

In principle there could also be approaches at a specifically immunological level as, for instance, by inducing an excess of 'blocking antibody' of the same specificity in a disease primarily involving T-immunocytes directed against a single tissue. Knowledge of the auto-antigens concerned is as yet inadequate to allow any practical approach along such lines, but the possibilities are worth discussion.

Possibilities of drug therapy

1. On general grounds an actively proliferating clone of cells is likely to be more sensitive to cytotoxic drugs like nitrogen mustard or cyclophosphamide than quiescent or less active clones. Cyclophosphamide and azathioprine appear to have some selectivity against immunocytes under specific stimulation and both drugs have been used with patchy success in SLE and other conditions in which the kidneys are involved. Azathioprine has also been used, usually in association with corticosteroids, in osteo-arthritis and active chronic hepatitis, in many cases with significant amelioration of symptoms. The disadvantage is that such drugs are variously toxic to many other

types of cells and are strongly suspect of increasing the probability of mutation of normal lymphoid cells to malignant or auto-immune character.

2. Cortisone, cortisol, and their various modifications are frequently highly effective in reducing acute phases of auto-immune conditions, so much so that when a clinical condition diagnosed as some form of auto-immune crisis fails to respond to an adequate dose of prednisone, the diagnosis should be reconsidered.

Cortisol is the main physiological glucocorticosteroid. It has a variety of striking effects when given in doses much larger than those circulating under natural conditions. Receptors responsive to the drug seem to be present on a very wide range of cells, but the effect produced is dependent on the nature of the cell and of the mammalian species being studied. The effects in clinical use point toward a specific capacity to damp down the effects of antigen–antibody union (or, more correctly, antigenic determinant/combining site union) where this involves the cell membrane of lymphoid cells. Such a view provides a satisfactory empirical basis on which to use the corticosteroids therapeutically, but it is probably far from being fully established or its mechanism understood.

The established effects of cortisol in the immunological field include: (1) a lymphocytolytic effect in large dose, involving mainly small lymphocytes and being particularly striking in the thymic cortex; (2) inhibition of antibody production but much more in rabbit, rat, and mouse than in guinea-pig, monkey, or man; (3) in contrast to (2), *in vitro* production of antibody by spleen fragments from a 'primed' rabbit *requires* about the physiological level of cortisol to be present in the culture tube; (4) inhibition of both delayed hypersensitivity and Arthus-type skin reactions; (5) anti-inflammatory effects including decrease in vascular permeability and exudation, with suppression of leucocytic migration.

Cortisol is one of the most important of the hormonal messengers responsible for adaptive changes in metabolism appropriate to immediate bodily needs. It may well have an important role in handling minor auto-immune episodes which probably occur frequently in all of us. Experience suggests that physiological production of cortisol is stimulated in acute auto-immune disease to as high a level as is compatible with balanced function. Administration of large doses of corticosteroids will frequently control severe symptoms in SLE or an acute exacerbation of rheumatoid arthritis, but prolonged administration can have disastrous effects elsewhere. These include bone rarefaction, suppression of adrenal function, diminished resistance to infections, notably tuberculosis, cataract of the eyes, peptic ulceration and perforation, psychotic changes and, finally, the full-blown Cushing's syndrome with 'moonface', acne, and failure of growth in children.

3. Often the only point in the pathogenic process that is accessible to therapeutic intervention is in relation to the tissue changes initiated by specific stimulation of auto-immunocytes of the T system. The effects are mediated by the liberation of lymphokines, pharmacologically active agents which produce what can be broadly called inflammatory effects. By far the greatest therapeutic effort against auto-immune disease comes in the treatment of the local pain and disability of rheumatoid arthritis and much effort has been spent in the development of anti-inflammatory drugs essentially on an empirical basis.

There seems to be general agreement that the simplest of all the minor analgesic drugs, aspirin (acetylsalicylic acid), remains the sheet anchor of routine treatment largely because of its relative freedom from unwanted effects. Phenylbutazone and indomethacin are more potent and considerably more productive of unpleasant or dangerous side-effects. With the recent increase in interest in the prostaglandins, a new approach to the anti-inflammatory drugs has come to light. It may become very important for both the understanding and control of inflammatory reactions that indomethacin, aspirin, and salicylates all inhibit the synthesis of prostaglandins E2 and F2A, the relative molar activity of the three drugs being 370:16:1 (Collier, 1971). The implication that prostaglandins are of special significance in the type of inflammation seen in rheumatoid arthritis is obvious and there will undoubtedly be a surge of new investigations in this area.

Two other widely used methods of treating rheumatoid arthritis, with gold compounds or with antimalarials such as chloroquine, appear to be wholly empirical.

Surgical intervention in auto-immune disease

If it is possible to eliminate an important, or the only, source of auto-immunogen without doing serious harm to the patient, surgery can have a part in the treatment of auto-immune disease. Splenectomy, thymectomy, and sub-total thyroidectomy have been used for the purpose.

Splenectomy has been used in the treatment of persisting auto-immune haemolytic anaemia and idiopathic thrombocytopenic purpura with a proportion of satisfactory results, particularly in idiopathic thrombocytopenic purpura. The rationale has usually been to allow the vulnerable elements, red cells or platelets, to survive longer in the circulation in functionally active form. There is, however, equally good reason to believe that in the process of breaking down effete or antibody-coated red cells or platelets, immunogenic material will be liberated and will be in higher concentration in the spleen than anywhere else. Proliferation of forbidden clones will probably be almost limited to the spleen. Splenectomy *should* be helpful in both conditions, but its success in practice will depend on the extent to which these activites are taking place in other lymphoid tissue as well.

The use of thymectomy in treating myasthenia gravis has been mentioned earlier without any serious attempt to inquire into its rationale. In line with our present approach it would be reasonable to assume that the significant source of auto-immunogen in myasthenia gravis is the myoid cells of the thymic medulla and that the characteristic germinal centres indicate local proliferation, presumably of B-immunocytes.

Also mentioned previously is the apparent success of thymectomy in three infants with severe auto-immune haemolytic anaemia. The only justification for venturing a hypothesis about what most haematologists would regard as a coincidence is to call for more study of the infantile thymus, which after all is at that time a major organ that may have some still unrecognized characteristics. The existence of ectopic cells (analogous to myoid cells) carrying a red cell surface antigen in some specially immunogenic form would bring the position into line with what has been postulated for myasthenia gravis.

Sub-total thyroidectomy, involving the removal of three-quarters or more of the gland, was, and to some extent still is, a standard treatment of Graves's disease, often with gratifying results. If the auto-immune etiology of the disease is accepted we must postulate that what surgery accomplished was a removal of most of the source of auto-immunogen. Assuming that the antigen corresponding to LATS is the receptor molecule which reacts with TSH, one could expect that more of this would be liberated in immunogenic form from an over-stimulated gland. A large reduction in the amount of thyroid tissue would then be a logical approach to cutting a vicious circle.

Approaches at the immunological level

The possibility of applying our understanding of tolerance to the treatment of auto-immune disease has often been raised, but, unless the use of immunosuppressive (cytotoxic) drugs such as azathioprine is included in the category, no practical applications have yet been claimed.

In essence, azathioprine is a convenient way of introducing the active agent 6-mercaptopurine (6-MP) into the body. The orthodox view of the action of 6-MP is that when it is given concomitantly with antigen it is incorporated into the nucleic acid of cells stimulated to proliferation by antigen and so renders such cells non-viable. The discovery by Schwartz and Dameshek in 1959 of this joint requirement of antigen and drug to produce tolerance was probably the first 'unexpected' pointer to the validity of the clonal selection concept. In so far as azathioprine or cyclophospamide have been effective in the treatment of auto-immune disease, this can be taken as supporting, in similar fashion, the forbidden clone extension of the concept.

There are, however, more directly immunological suggestions that have been raised. In discussing them I shall necessarily assume that the views in regard to the pathogenesis of auto-immune disease that have been adopted are correct. This may necessitate modification in the formulation of some suggestions from their original form. There seem to be four theoretical possibilities:

1. To administer auto-antigen in a tolerigenic form.

2. To induce the production of blocking antibody to inhibit T-cell activity.

3. To induce a specific immune attack on auto-immunocytes, assuming that these are antigenically distinguishable from normal immunocytes.

4. To disturb pharmacologically the balance between proliferative and destructive responses to specific contact with antigen.

Before saying something about each of these possibilities, it must be emphasized that almost all will depend on the identification and isolation of the relevant auto-antigens. So far there has been extremely little work at the molecular level in this field and any soundly based attempts at clinical use of any of the methods will have to await new experimental developments. One would expect the New Zealand mice to provide the first opportunities for the experimental work.

1. Irrespective of how a cell becomes tolerant, whether by its physical elimination from the body, sterile activation, or functional inhibition, a given antigen can often be presented in forms which are prone to provoke tolerance and in others that stimulate a proliferative response. In broad terms the polymerized form of *Salmonella* flagellin is highly immunogenic in rats compared to the monomer. The monomer is, however, much more tolerigenic than the polymer. Another example that is possibly more relevant is the immunogenicity of a slightly denatured preparation of bovine gammaglobulin in mice and the tolerigenic action of the same antigen carefully freed of all aggregated material.

The possibility would always be present that a clone of immunocytes had auto-immune qualities *because* it was resistant to any tolerigenic action of these sorts. One would expect, however, that the differences from normal were quantitative and that raising the concentration of the tolerigenic material might be effective.

2. There is a hint from the frequency of arthritis in agammaglobulinemics that antibody may have an important damping effect on any auto-immune process mediated by T-immunocytes. Unfortunately very little is known about the relative immunogenicity of auto-antigens for T and B immune systems. There may well be differences from one individual to another and there are certainly differences between species (cf. guinea-pig and rat, for instance). The possibility that a patient with Hashimoto's disease but no circulating antibody would be improved by a series of intravenous injections of semi-purified thyroid microsomal antigen to provoke an antibody response may one day be put to practical test.

3. Lymphocytes have an undoubtedly wide range of antigenic determinants on their surfaces and it is not impossible that each auto-immune clone has a specific antigen related to its pathogenic character. None such have been detected and it is therefore rather pointless to go further and think of the possibility that there may be a common new antigen in all the forbidden clones of a given patient. In view, however, of the extensive current knowledge of surface antigenic determinants in mouse lymphocytes, there seems to be good reason for undertaking a specific

study of the point in NZB mice. There would be one outstanding difficulty, viz. that there is no syngeneic strain of NZB lacking only the capacity to develop auto-immune haemolytic anaemia, which could be used to develop specific antisera against the hypothetical 'auto-immune' antigen.

4. In discussing the 'phenocopies' of auto-immune disease that have followed prolonged use of certain drugs in man, particularly α-methyldopa (mimicking AHA) and procainamide with its SLE-like symptoms, it was suggested that the drug might change the micro-environment where immunocyte and auto-antigen interacted, so that the balance between elimination and proliferation was tipped in the latter direction. The mechanism of this postulated effect is unknown and the discovery of such drugs has always been unpredictable. Their existence, however, does raise the possibility that extensive screening tests might equally empirically bring to light drugs with an opposite effect, in, as it were, bringing the disturbed balance of an auto-immunocyte back to the normal equilibrium point. Once again the New Zealand mice could, with some experimental ingenuity, be used for such a screening programme.

None of these four approaches seem at all likely to find clinical applications, but one does feel that a more whole-hearted approach to understanding the basic pathogenesis of the NZB mouse disease, plus the therapeutic experiments called for as understanding increased, might open up some more promising approach than any now visible.

Conclusion

As one goes over the clinical accounts of severe auto-immune disease it is hard to avoid feeling that extremely little has been accomplished, and that if there is ever to be an effective treatment of auto-immune disease some wholly new approach will need to be discovered in the future. It may be salutary to think of the various forms of treatment for tuberculosis that were current before 1945. Artificial pneumothorax was then standard treatment and clinicians were sure of its beneficial effects. I remember well being very unpopular for claiming in a lecture given in 1945 that there was no evidence of any improvement in the results over the last twenty years and that 'something somewhere is wrong and it is incumbent on those concerned with the treatment of tuberculosis to remedy it' (Burnet, 1946). When streptomycin, isoniazid, and PAS came a few years later, collapse therapy vanished almost overnight.

I am not optimistic that anything equivalent will emerge to produce a similar change in the handling of auto-immune disease. For the present I can only express the same sort of scepticism that I voiced about collapse therapy for tuberculosis twenty-seven years ago. A seriously ill patient must be treated and there are conscientious clinicians who are convinced that careful use of a combination of corticosteroids and azathioprine in doses small enough to avoid the unwanted side-effects can control a condition such as chronic active hepatitis for long periods and allow the patient to lead an active life. Any form of prolonged therapy for an auto-immune condition must obviously be handled according to the patient's response and requires frequent assessment of all the serological and haematological criteria that are relevant. Undoubtedly corticosteroids must be used in critical situations, but, unless very efficient clinical and laboratory surveillance can be maintained, prolonged use of corticosteroids and cytotoxic drugs presents a considerable hazard of iatrogenic disease. There is much to be said for a thorough test of aspirin in suitable form and dosage as maintenance therapy before using the more potent and more dangerous drugs.

There are, of course, many aspects of the various auto-immune diseases that call for skilful treatment quite unrelated to immunological and inflammatory aspects. Replacement therapy for hormone lack is the most important in thyroid, adrenal or parathyroid disease, and in pernicious anaemia. In all the crippling joint diseases the amelioration of physical disability by physiotherapy or surgery is important. There are many other aspects of needed medical care, but none of them are relevant to the purpose of this book.

CHAPTER 14

The significance of auto-immunity for ageing

With the rapidly expanding population of old people in every affluent country, important new social problems are emerging. It is natural, therefore, that gerontology is attracting many of the academically minded, and within the medical profession a fully fledged speciality of geriatrics is growing up. With age every bodily system becomes less efficient and more vulnerable, though in some the effect is more striking than in others. Anyone interested in almost any aspect of human biology will find that some facet of ageing is relevant to his field of study. Immunologists are no exception and in any recent discussion on theories of ageing the auto-immune or immunological approach will be found mentioned. It is characteristic of theorizing in any difficult biological area not susceptible to effective experimental study that the three formulations of immunological approaches to ageing, by Walford, Burch, and myself, have not very much in common. There is a great deal more to ageing than the development of low-grade auto-immune disease, but this is part of the story and it would be inappropriate to omit the topic in a book on general aspects of auto-immunity.

The biology of ageing

Any approach to ageing as a biological phenomenon must start with the recognition that the length of life-span is an intrinsic characteristic of every species of organism that is subject to natural death. Amongst the mammals senile changes are found at 2 years in a mouse, 3 in a rat, 12–14 in a large dog, 30 in a horse, 70 in a man. In each species there is a wide scatter around those values, but the general picture is unmistakable. In every animal, including man, there is a biological clock, wound up at conception, which rules the tempo and periodicity of his functioning and runs down around a predetermined date. The ultimate problem of ageing is to determine the nature of that clock.

Subject to the qualification that we may be omitting something of unrecognized importance, the significant changes with age in man and probably all mammals are as follows.

First the physical changes: greying of hair, loss of teeth, atrophy and wrinkling of the skin, bone fragility. The last two are associated with and probably due to atrophy and diminished strength and elasticity of the collagen fibres of the body.

Progressive reduction of the lymphoid system with a conspicuously early atrophy of the thymus.

Increasing inefficiency of immunological function as shown by the steady rise in mortality from non-specific or previously unencountered specific infections with age.

An increase in signs of somatic mutation in the skin and a rapidly increasing susceptibility to malignant disease and several forms of auto-immune disease.

Probably the most suitable summing-up of old age in man is to express the process as an increasing vulnerability to every sort of hazard. In a sense there may be no such thing as natural death, only death resulting from some accidental happening that to a younger individual would be trivial.

It has been central to all my discussion of antibody production, malignant disease, and auto-immune disease in the last fifteen years that all somatic cells are subject to mutational change. Probably everyone who has thought about ageing will agree that there must be an accumulation of cellular 'impairments' throughout life. Any mutation, whether a simple point change in a nucleotide or some more complex deletion or rearrangement of genetic material, will in almost every instance diminish the functional effectiveness of the cell. Mutant cells will either be so abnormal as to provoke a reaction that will eliminate them or they will persist in a sub-functional state, remaining potentially susceptible to sequential mutation of other types. Having regard to the number of cells in the human body and the fact that mutation can occur in resting as well as in proliferating cells, there must be a steady and accelerating increase in the proportion of poorly functioning cells in the body. This will be largely due to the accumulation of multiple (sequential) mutations in the same cell line. It may be remembered that Burch found that the age-specific incidence curve for fracture of the neck of the femur in women corresponded to a coincidence of seven distinct random events. The standard curve for age incidence of cancer is usually interpreted as due to a series of at least two sequential mutations, with the earlier one or ones providing a proliferative advantage over unmutated cells so that a population of the primary mutant can be built up within which a second or later mutation of the necessary type may occur. Similarly, the approach that both Burch and I have used to auto-immune disease ascribes the appearance of pathogenic immunocytes (or forbidden clones) to somatic mutation often in more than one cell line.

In a broad sense there is no alternative to the view that some, many, or all of the phenomena of ageing are based on the occurrence of somatic mutation and secondary results thereof. This, however, is a very incomplete answer and does not, for instance, throw any light whatever on why a mouse ages some 35–50 times faster than a man. So far there is no accepted answer to that question in any other terms than evolutionary ones. For a wild mouse, a life-span of something just over a year in relation to its ecology and reproductive performance gives the optimal conditions for survival of the species. Foı human beings, 45–50 years (to the end of reproductive life), plus another 15 or 20 years to bring up the last offspring, brings us close to the allotted span. Those explanations provide no hints as to the biochemical or cellular mechanisms which are concerned.

Limits to cell proliferation

Like many others, I have been impressed (sometimes, I think, against my better judgement) with the idea that the Hayflick limit may contain the clue to the nature of the biological clock, which says how long a man or a mouse may live if he avoids mischance. Hayflick observed that cell cultures initiated from human embryo lung and maintained under optimal conditions would proliferate as fibroblasts with the normal (euploid) complement of chromosomes for many generations but not indefinitely. Proliferation faded out and finally ceased at around the 50th cell generation (38th to 64th in one set of experiments). If the cells underwent mutation, a continuing line which like the standard HeLa cells of the laboratory could proliferate indefinitely might appear, but in Hayflick's experience all such lines were aneuploid, with chromosomal abnormalities of number or form. Cell culture is far from equivalent to the activities of cells *in vivo* and there may be no better reason for the Hayflick limit than inability to provide some unrecognized component of the medium.

Nevertheless it is attractive to consider the possibility that, once a cell at some early stage of development has passed the point at which it could still give rise to a germ line descendant cell, it accepts an intrinsic limitation in the number of possible divisions its descendant line can undergo. Many lines in the course of their differentiation reach a stage after which no further mitosis can occur. These are post-mitotic or end cells. If we confine ourselves to the cell lines that interest immunologists, two such examples of cells that have reached a physiological post-mitotic stage are the mature plasma cell and the mast cell. Once an immunoblast has been set into activity along the plasmacyte sequence, mitosis ceases after about eight or nine divisions. This appears to be a result of an inbuilt genetic programme. Very rarely that maturation programme is cancelled by somatic mutation, and, virtually without any change in functional capacity, the plasmablast continues to multiply indefinitely, giving rise to the semi-malignant condition of multiple myelomatosis.

It would not seem biologically absurd that for cells which do not require specific functional development to post-mitotics, the turning-off mechanism should be made use of to determine the programming of the life span. In 1970 I suggested that this may apply to the stem cell lines in the bone marrow from which circulating lymphocytes and plasma cells are derived. It is by no means excluded that this holds also for stem lines from which fibroblasts, monocytes and their derivatives, and granulocytes descend, but my primary interests were on cells of immunological potentialities. If to Hayflick's 50 generations we add another 20 to cover the period from the zygote to the standard embryo used to start the cell cultures, the 'real' limit becomes 70 cell generations. This allows the production of $2^{70} = 10^{21}$ cells, which is more than adequate to cover all the cells ever having an existence in the body of a 70-year-old man.

If the Hayflick limit is going to function as the life-span controller, it is obvious that it must do so because some cell line necessary to life uses up its allotted generations more rapidly than any other essential line. In looking over the possibilities for the controlling cell type, there is one outstanding clue. In every type of vertebrate, and conspicuously so in mammals, the thymus, a major element in the development of the immune system, atrophies early and is always functionally insignificant in old age. The other primary immunocyte producer, known as a specific organ only in birds (bursa of Fabricius), also atrophies early in life. The possibility that the lymphocytes of the immune system, particularly those derived from the thymus (T-immunocytes), were directly concerned in the ageing process seemed worth exploring.

In mammals, including man, the thymus, at least in the young animal, has a more active cell turnover than any other organ. The population changes completely in twenty days in the cortex of the mouse thymus. There is evidence that the 'store of generations' is being used up even more rapidly than this would indicate. Many pyknotic nuclei indicative of cell death are always to be seen in the cortex, and Metcalf calculates that at least 95 per cent of the lymphocytes produced in the thymus of the mouse at 6–12 weeks of age are rapidly destroyed. I have suggested that this destruction is of newly differentiated immunocytes reactive with 'self' components. Further, it is well known to clinical and experimental pathologists that any infection or other stress results in massive destruction of thymocytes, followed by a heavy call for restocking, presumably from the bone marrow. It would be a reasonable deduction from the Hayflick hypothesis, which we are exploring, that the progressive atrophy of the thymus from adolescence onwards is due to a growing scarcity of stem cells of the necessary type and with enough 'spare generations' to complete their intrathymic proliferation and differentiation to immunocytes. By analogy both with the mammalian thymus and the avian bursa it seems highly probable that the centres of primary B-cell differentiation behave similarly to the thymus. Certainly the capacity to produce new antibodies diminishes greatly in old age.

The question now arises as to whether a credible case can be made for regarding a progressive loss of immunological function as the central 'rate-determining' feature of ageing. There is no doubt whatever that all immune responses do weaken with age, but then so do virtually all other physiological functions. The alternatives to be examined are whether (1) immunological fade-out is just one of a whole series of progressive changes involving nearly every function in parallel fashion, or (2) many or most of the other changes are secondary to the early development of immunological weakness which results from exhaustion of 'available generations' in the stem cell lines of the immune system. Throughout the discussion the point to be borne in mind is that any answer must be directed primarily toward explaining why natural life-span is a specific characteristic of each species and can range in mammals from one year to a hundred years; yet the signs of old age are basically similar in each species.

We can start by recapitulating the more important signs of old age in mammals, in addition to a general reduction in activity and functional activity plus an increased vulnerability to almost any impact from the environment. They are: (1) atrophy of connective and fibrous tissues associated with decrease in amount and chemical change (cross-linkage) in collagen fibres; (2) widespread degenerative changes in the smaller blood vessels; (3) rapidly increasing incidence of malignant tumours and of skin blemishes, benign tumours, and other expressions of somatic mutation; (4) increasing vulnerability to non-specific respiratory or intestinal infections and to any specific infectious diseases not previously experienced; (5) greying of the hair which in some strains of horses and in some human individuals appears to occur quite independently of the other signs of ageing and will be excluded from the discussion.

If the immune system, and particularly thymus-dependent immunocytes, are significantly concerned in holding back the onset of ageing, their action must be mediated very largely through the function of immunological surveillance. This has been mentioned briefly in Chapter 3 and reviewed extensively elsewhere, but here something more must be said about the possible bearing of the immunological control function (surveillance) on auto-immune processes.

Immunological surveillance in relation to auto-immune disease

Most malignant tumours, human and experimental, manifest antigenic determinants not carried by the cells they arise from. Some of the antigens, particularly in guinea-pigs, are relatively 'strong'. A tumour administered as living cells intradermally can produce short-lasting local lesions which provoke a cytotoxic response eliminating the tumours and leaving the animal immune to the normally lethal challenge of an intramuscular injection of tumour cells of the same strain. Other experimental tumours have only weak antigenicity in syngeneic hosts and some have no detectable capacity to immunize.

The most cogent evidence of the importance of immunological surveillance in man is the strikingly increased incidence of malignant tumours in children with immunodeficiency diseases and in patients who have received renal transplants and been subsequently maintained on immunosuppressive therapy. It is of special interest in relation to our present theme that more than half the tumours in both groups are derived from lymphoid cells, most being recitulum cell sarcomas or lymphomas. In the cases arising in patients under continuing treatment with immunosuppressive drugs there is an unusual incidence of such tumours in the brain.

The incidence of malignant disease in relation to age will depend essentially on the interaction of two stochastic processes: the accumulation of somatic mutations with proliferative advantage till a malignant clone emerges whose potential antigenicity may range from zero to 'strong', and the development of clones of T-immunocytes of sufficient activity to deal with a nidus of malignant cells. If this is correct it should follow that tumours of significant antigenicity, i.e. carrying antigenic determinants distinctively different from any normally accessible in the body, are likely to be cut short and never reach clinical visibility if they arise in early or middle life. Conversely, tumours arising in young people will be expected to be non-antigenic and of correspondingly greater malignancy. It should also follow that when T-immunocyte activity is damped down by azathioprine and other immunosuppressive drugs, any tumour which appears in exceptional numbers should be of a type that in the normal individual is readily eliminated by the surveillance process.

There is other evidence that lymphocytic cells carry relatively numerous antigens on their surface and that some of these change with the development of malignant activity (Old and Boyse). As yet there does not appear to be any direct evidence that an auto-immune clone of lymphocytes has an antigenic determinant directly associated with its auto-immune capacity, but one feels that with the present active interest in cell membrane proteins there should be no insuperable difficulty in devising experimental approaches to test for the presence of such determinants. It is known that Burkitt lymphoma cells (*a*) are immunocytes in the sense of liberating immunoglobulin in culture and (*b*) have specific antigens capable of inducing delayed hypersensitivity (by skin test) in the host individual. Idiotypic antibodies, specific for a single myeloma protein, are well known and it is by no means inconceivable that the appearance of an exceptionally large clone of uniform T-immunocytes might initiate an immune response directed against the specific receptor as antigen. For reasons discussed earlier the casual appearance of auto-immune clones must be a common occurrence, and an essential part of the fail-safe mechanisms for inhibiting or eliminating them could well be by the exercise of the surveillance function. Nearly all auto-immune conditions are subject to remission. It is stated as a clinical impression that a first episode of rheumatoid arthritis coming on acutely and intensely is considerably more likely to be followed by a prolonged or permanent remission than one which develops insidiously. This suggests the rapid build-up of a pathogenic clone and its subsequent elimination by a surveillance-type immune response.

It is not likely that a diffuse scattering of somatic mutant cells with some antigenic change throughout the tissues would ever induce an immune response. Only when there is a significant local region of proliferation will this be at all likely. The situation where immunocytes are concerned is quite different, since any significant auto-immune activity will necessarily involve the development of a large uniform population of immunocytes which, if they are antigenic at all, will have uniform antigenicity. An immune response, probably essentially of T-cells, will in most cases be effective and provides the simplest explanation of remissions in auto-immune disease. Reactions of this sort, which virtually postulate a state of civil war between lymphocyte populations in lymphoid tissue and in circulation, may sound confusing, but there is nothing to veto the hypothesis. In some ways the situation in rheumatoid arthritis, where antibodies are being formed against antibody serving as antigen, is analogous.

To paraphrase slightly a previous discussion of this point, the concept of T-cell-based surveillance of aberrant lymphocytic populations conforms with and illuminates a wide variety of clinical and experimental phenomena. These include, in addition to the frequency of lymphoreticular neoplasms under prolonged immunosuppression or in immunological deficiency diseases, the frequency of lymphomatous diseases in mice and men, the extreme difficulty in interpreting the histopathology of lymph nodes and the frequency with which frank auto-immune disease occurs as a terminal feature of chronic leukaemia or Hodgkin's disease. It may also be highly relevant to the pathogenesis of infectious mononucleosis and its not infrequent association with a benign auto-immune haemolytic anaemia.

The primary and secondary results of somatic mutation in relation to ageing

The general thesis that is emerging in regard to ageing can perhaps be summarized in the briefest possible form as:

1. There are genetic limits to the number of generations of somatic cell proliferation *in vivo* as well as *in vitro*.

2. Somatic mutation continues through life with progressive accumulation of cells carrying one or more mutations, mostly with some impairment of function.

3. The effectiveness of all immune responses diminishes steadily with age.

It still remains to bring these three factors into relationship with one another.

If, as has been postulated, the Hayflick limit has its effect in relation to the stem cell lines via the thymus and the lymphoid tissue generally, there is a valid reason why immunological effectiveness should weaken in old age. The main weakness may well be an inability to provide the diversity of immune patterns which in a young animal ensures that any type of specific response that is needed can be mounted.

Somatic mutation occurs probably at a fairly uniform rate in all tissues throughout life. This must result in an accumulating impairment of function, but the rate of mutation would be inadequate to account for the observed extent of senile changes.

One important consequence of somatic mutation for ageing is, of course, the appearance of benign or malignant tumours, usually by a sequence of mutations increasing proliferative capacity in any way. This, however, has no bearing on the generalized tissue damage and degeneration of old age. Some means by which widespread damage involving whole systems can be derived from relatively few primary somatic mutations is required. Two such mechanisms are suggested.

The first depends on the fact that as soon as a clone of pathogenic auto-immunocytes has become viable, it can expand indefinitely under the stimulus of contact with the corresponding auto-antigen. Irrespective of whether T-cells or antibody is responsible for the damaging effect, either can, in principle, reach all the cells in the body that are susceptible to damage.

The second possibility is, so far, only a speculation. It is possible in principle for a clone of T-immunocytes to arise which is specifically directed against a 'new' antigen arising by somatic mutation in a considerable number of cells. Reaction against individual cells, if they were widely dispersed, might produce so many foci of damage involving adjacent cells, as well as the specific target cells, that the over-all result could resemble an auto-immune attack on the system concerned.

Obviously there is immense scope for damage, but from the immunological angle there are consequences to be considered from the postulated exhaustion of stem cells from which new immune patterns can emerge. There will be little response in the aged to the appearance of non-malignant but potentially antigenic somatic mutations, just as the response to malignancy is absent or ineffective. By the time old age is reached, most of those genetically susceptible to some auto-immune diseases, like SLE or thyrotoxicosis, will have been eliminated. For those who survive and become progressively subject to the disabilities of age the possibility of developing some form of auto-immune disease will remain. The process or sequence of processes by which a final somatic mutation produces a potential initiation of a pathogenic clone will continue, though with a progressively diminishing frequency. The possibility too will remain that a potential initiator produced long before and surviving as a 'long-lived lymphocyte' may find conditions suitable for its activation. At the same time the capacity to confront and deal with anomalous cells will be progressively weakening. What may be much more important in relation both to auto-immune and malignant disease is the inability of the exhausted T system to produce the necessary new patterns of surveillance cell receptors.

Some additional aspects of the ageing process need to be looked at in the light of this general hypothesis of accumulating somatic mutations and the immunological reactions to which they give rise.

Hardin Jones in 1959 presented a compelling case for looking at the Makeham–Gompertz exponential curve of mortality in man as a self-accelerating process. As he put it, any 'impairment' of bodily function increases the likelihood of subsequent impairment. Hardship and heavy incidence of disease in a youthful community meant, in his view, a shortened life-span of those so exposed. Life in Japanese prison camps of south-east Asia in the Second World War had already had a visible effect on the life expectation of those who came out. By his nomenclature, impairment resulted when any environmental impact, any stress, pushed a bodily system beyond the limits of rapid physiological recovery. In common-sense terms of the conventional wisdom of the community this is merely a statement that a healthy life free from physical or emotional stress and from serious illness is conducive to longevity. If the essential physiological effect of stress is to quicken the rate at which cells are turned over and in large part destroyed in the thymus, the relation to life-span is immediately explicable. It is not easy to see any alternative explanation with the same simple relevance to the facts.

The progressive reduction of and chemical change in collagen with age is seen in all mammalian species and in man appears to be directly responsible for such features as the thinning and wrinkling of the skin and in large part for the weakening of the bones in old age. No satisfactory explanation has been given to cover the facts that collagen is chemically similar in all mammals, that the changes with age are also broadly similar but the time-scale so different. It cannot possibly be a chemical process due to something called 'wear and tear', and its origin must be sought in cellular and genetic processes. The origin of the active proliferating fibroblasts which are responsible for collagen synthesis has not been resolved. Most studies have been made in relation to the development of fibroblasts and collagen in areas of inflammation and repair. There are suggestions that in such regions fibroblasts arise from activation of local connective tissue cells, from lymphocytes entering the area from the circulation or from monocytes also brought by the blood. After reading recent reviews on the inflammatory process one ends by wondering whether all three processes may not occur. There is at least no decisive objection to the view that the fibroblast derives in one way or another from the bone marrow stem cells rather than wholly from cells descending consistently from the first mesenchymal cells in each local area. New technical approaches may necessitate a change of opinion, but at the present time I believe the stem cell origin via the circulation is justified.

It was once common to include many of the auto-immune diseases under the term collagen diseases. This appears to have been based on the inflammatory processes which often seemed to involve connective tissues and, of necessity, the predominant protein collagen in such situations. It is extremely unlikely that collagen itself would ever serve as an auto-antibody nor is there any suggestion that fibroblasts are ever the specific target cells of an auto-immune process. There is, in fact, virtually no clear indication of what is responsible for the loss and chemical modification of collagen which is characteristic of old age. Clearly, complex synthetic processes are involved, subject to availability of cells and the competence of the enzymes and other elements involved in the formation and spatial laying down of collagen. Exhaustion of the supply of stem cells and accumulation of mutational errors is perhaps the most likely origin of the degeneration of collagen in old age. It is a concept that is conformable with the Hayflick limit approach, but there is no positive evidence to support it. I can see no hint that auto-immune processes are concerned.

CHAPTER 15

A programme for the future

On comparing what I have written in this book with what clinicians and immunologists are currently writing, I find that I am still swimming strongly against the stream. It is not that there are well-organized and argued rival interpretations but rather a general disinclination to go beyond the observable findings. In medicine a theoretical interpretation that gives no lead to effective prevention or treatment has no practical significance. Most writers, when forced by convention to make some remarks on etiology, produce a limited discussion on auto-antibodies, essentially from the old instructive standpoint. Few have so far discussed the role of the T-immune system and there is generally an implicit suggestion that an acceptable 'cause' for each important condition will eventually be found; most probably a slow virus.

The view that this negative approach is unjustified has been laid out to the best of my ability in this book and it rests with the future to accept the forbidden clone approach in some progressively modifiable form or replace it with something more satisfactory. Conceivably there are experiments or observations to be made which will be incompatible with the forbidden clone approach. The history of every major biological controversy of the past, however, suggests that when new facts emerge they will favour a broad Darwinian interpretation of auto-immune disease that will develop naturally out of the present outline. This has happened or is happening at the expense of simpler, more obvious doctrines of organic evolution, of adaptation in micro-organisms, of antibody production, and of cancer.

No set of scientific generalizations can ever be more than temporary. Future discoveries will certainly require progressive modification of the ideas and the therapeutic practices of today. When an understanding of disease offers no logical and practicable approach to prevention or cure, as appears to be the case with all serious types of auto-immune disease, it becomes of special urgency to consider the direction of future research. Are there any chances that some new approach will offer practical benefit or any extensions of the forbidden clone hypothesis which call for new investigations?

In the light of the foregoing chapters it seems appropriate to end, and in a sense to epitomize, the approach by discussing some possibilities for future research. They can be placed under five headings, the first two being concerned with genetic predisposition to auto-immune conditions, the third and fourth with the nature of the processes seen clinically, and the fifth with further exploitation of animal models.

Population genetics of auto-immune disease

Genetic investigations of human disease conditions which are not clearly concerned with a single gene difference are notoriously difficult. The most that can be said in regard to the inheritance of auto-immune conditions is that the great majority of investigations have shown that first-degree relatives of index patients with almost any of the standard auto-immune diseases will differ from similar relatives of an appropriately matched 'normal control group' in showing:

1. A significantly greater incidence of signs and symptoms conventionally associated with auto-immune disease, not necessarily the same disease as the index cases.

2. A significantly higher incidence of the commonly tested auto-antibodies: rheumatoid factor, antinuclear factor, thyroid auto-antibody, and gastric parietal cell antibody.

In addition, there are families on record where gross immunological anomalies such as agammaglobulinaemia and a variety of auto-immune diseases and haematological abnormalities seem to be associated.

It seems to be reasonably certain that there are some genetic factors that predispose generally to auto-immune disease and the possibility that certain combinations may strongly predispose to a particular disease, for example, SLE, is far from being excluded. The fact that when mice of a pure line subject to haemolytic anaemia are mated with an apparently normal line from the same original stock all the females and most of the males amongst the F1 progeny show an SLE-like disease provides a good indication of the sort of co-operation of genes to be expected in human populations.

There are, however, no pure lines of human beings and identical twins are not of much use for the investigation of rare conditions or for any analysis beyond a simple statement that genetic factors do or do not play a dominant role. In principle the only socially practical way to obtain comprehensive medical-genetic information is to record the descent, verified by the standard blood group checks, of all individuals in a large, relatively stable population for several generations. If physical characteristics, major illnesses, and all medically significant anomalies were accurately recorded, modern computer techniques could probably sort out the rules of inheritance of auto-immune disease and many other conditions.

If the current civilization and its computers survive the crisis-catastrophe that most of us fear within the next fifty years, such studies may become essential. They would be strongly resisted in English-speaking countries at the present time and state-wide organization of medical and genetic 'databanks' would be politically unthinkable. One doubts, however, whether anything less would within a hundred years elucidate the inheritance of auto-immune disease or provide what will sooner or later be urgently needed: the scientific data on which rational eugenic policies may eventually be based.

Immunological vigour as a genetic factor

Before discussing the potentialities of direct cloning and study of pure lines of immunocytes in culture, some thought may be given to the question that has been raised in regard to the New Zealand mice. Is it possible that the genetic character of immunological vigour or resistance to the development of tolerance which is observed in NZB mice plays a part in human predisposition to auto-immune disease?

Scattered through the literature one finds statements that in addition to most patients with gross auto-immune disease a significant proportion of their first degree relatives show hypergammaglobulinaemia, i.e. an abnormally high level of immunoglobulins in the blood. It seems to be a real possibility that this may often be an indication of predisposition to auto-immune disease, and that specific research on this aspect could be practical. On the NZ mice analogy, hypergammaglobulinaemia could indicate that to maintain the normal feedback control that prevents over-production of any one type of antibody a considerably higher concentration is required. It would be of obvious interest to know the distribution of immune specificities in such people, but at present there seems to be no practical approach. It could be of real value, however, to make periodical bleedings from a group of people with high immunoglobulin levels and store serum for subsequent study when any of them developed overt auto-immune disease.

With the developments of laboratory methods for demonstrating *in-vitro* induction of antibody formation and with larger doses of antigen, immune paralysis (Diener and Armstrong, 1969), it may become possible to apply similar methods to human material from lymph node biopsies or even perhaps with a concentrated population of blood lymphocytes. With the NZB results in mind, one might expect a higher level of antigen concentration would be needed to induce the change from antibody production to paralysis in auto-immune subjects than in normal individuals. As in the mouse experiments, standard antigens, perhaps *Salmonella* flagellin and bovine gammaglobulin, would be used.

In-vitro *cloning of immunocytes*

Laboratory investigation of developed auto-immune disease does not as a rule go beyond testing for the well-known types of auto-antibody and following the titres of any that are found to be present. Studies of the specific character of immunocytes has hardly begun; but it is clearly along such lines that any experimental implications of the forbidden clone concept must be looked for.

Some of these have already been mentioned, but one feels that current developments in experimental cytology are rapidly bringing the possibilities of direct study of pathogenic clones of human cells into the realm of actuality. Warm type auto-immune haemolytic anaemia obviously offers the most promising material, particularly since splenectomy and, in infants, thymectomy are still acceptable approaches to treatment. In view of the standardization of Jerne's methods for enumerating plaque-forming cells (PFC) and of the success of Wilson's, Holmes's, and Warner's work on NZB mice, it should be relatively easy to devise a method applicable to clinical material. No doubt results will initially be harder to obtain and interpret than with

PFC producing a standard antibody against a foreign red cell, but the difficulties should only be technical ones.

Leddy and Bakemeier (1965) have already produced presumptive evidence that the antibody eluted from Coombs positive cells in AHA is monoclonal in origin. Once methods of cloning immunocytes *in vitro* have been established, other markers could be applied to assess the probable number of pathogenic clones concerned. The use of G6PD isozymes as markers in female heterozygotes has been very useful in cancer studies and no doubt this and analogous methods will eventually be applied in immunopathological work. The erythrocyte is such a satisfactory target cell that it seems hardly worth while choosing any other disease than AHA for detailed investigation along these lines at the present time.

There are many clones of immunoglobulin-producing human cells maintained in culture at the present time, but there are suggestions that they cannot be so maintained in normal physiological function. Some lines, for instance, produce more than one type of immunoglobulin. Obviously the improvement of culture methods and their application to a wide range of immunological and immunopathological situations is the most promising corner of immunology at the present time. A short cut to the study of auto-immune cell clones might be to obtain myeloma cells in culture from one of the not very uncommon cases of monoclonal macroglobulinaemia in which the abnormal globulin has the character of rheumatoid factor.

There is still nothing equivalent to multiple myeloma (a monoclonal proliferation of a mutant B-cell) known for the T system, but unless all our ideas are wrong there must be a variety of lymphomatous tumours which are monoclonal and derived from a T-immunocyte. Sooner or later techniques for cloning such cells in culture and identifying the immunological characteristics of the line will be developed.

At the clinical level we are just beginning to find appropriate laboratory approaches to the T-immune system. Skin tests giving delayed hypersensitivity type reactions will probably remain as an essential first approach. Stimulation of circulating lymphocytes to blast transformation by antigen and the production of migration inhibiting factor are still topics for the research laboratory rather than routine clinical procedures, but they may be expected to develop in that direction. For all tests designed to demonstrate directly or indirectly the presence of T-cells of specific character, the most important need is probably to provide relatively pure, active, and sterile preparations of the auto-antigen in question.

So far, most of the possibilities discussed are as applicable to physiologically normal immunocytes as to those concerned with auto-immunity. It is probable that most immunologists, if pressed, would predict that 'auto-immunocytes', once cloned and characterized, would not fall outside the range of the heterogeneous population of immunocytes found in normal individuals. The forbidden clone hypothesis will only stand in its current form if auto-immune, semi-malignant (chronic lymphatic leukaemia perhaps), and malignant clones of immunocytes can be experimentally differentiated from normal clones of cultured lymphocytes with immunologically defined function.

From both academic and practical angles the most promising line of differentiation would be in regard to cell surface antigens. At present this seems to be impossible in principle in the absence of syngeneic providers of the necessary antisera. Nevertheless, some interesting progress is being made in studying the behaviour of the patient's own serum and lymphocytes against cultured cells from his surgically removed cancer. Out of such work there could well develop ways of identifying immune responses against mutant antigens in lymphocytes that were relevant to their pathogenic activity. It is unlikely, but perhaps not impossible, that the development of auto-immune capacity was associated with one or a small number of new antigenic determinants on the cell surface. If that were once established, we might at last have a glimmer of hope of developing a specific therapy.

In the field of localized auto-immune disease probably the most urgent academic requirement is to identify the nature of the immunocytes associated with infiltration and germinal centre development in the target organ. What observations have been published are consistent with some at least of them being specific auto-immunocytes, but probably none of the experiments would withstand a modern critical appraisal. There should surely be ways by which the cells in a germinal centre of Hashimoto's disease can be identified as to their immunological function.

Further work on the New Zealand mice

I have made much use of results with the New Zealand mice in developing the general approach to auto-immune disease that characterizes this book. Like most others who have worked with them, I regard NZB and NZB/W as providing true models of human auto-immune disease. As such they must obviously be even more intensively studied than they have been.

Long-term genetic studies may well be the most important. If, as everything suggests, the quality is a polygenic one, there would seem to be promise of fruitful results in screening large numbers of F2 hybrids of the primary B/W and B/C matings for relevant qualities and developing new pure lines of any combinations that seem promising. In view of the value that genetic anomalies involving the immune system in man have been in immunology (for example, in defining the T and B systems), a genetic analysis of the components of the auto-immune haemolytic anaemia of NZB and the SLE-like glomerulonephritis of NZB/W could not fail to be enlightening.

Almost equally interesting would be an extension of the work already well begun by Warner and his collaborators on the allotypes involved in the auto-antibodies coating red cells in NZB hybrids with mice of different globulin allotypes and the implications of the results for the nature of the auto-immune process.

It should be kept in mind that if the hypothesis derived from a fusion of the forbidden clone concept with Burch's calculations of the number of somatic mutations needed to initiate auto-immune disease is correct, it might become possible to 'synthesize' genetically strains in which all but one of the necessary mutations is fixed in the germ line. Such mice should regularly develop disease at an early age. As in all experimental work, the most significant discoveries will be those which cannot be forecast. I feel confident that there are phases of the fail-safe system of dealing with the accidental appearance of forbidden clones which have not yet been recognized. A well-balanced genetic cyto-genetic and immunochemical attack on the New Zealand mice may well be one of the most rewarding prospects of future immunology.

A final summary

Since 1957 I have been consistently supporting the opinion that malignant disease, antibody production, and auto-immune disease can only be interpreted as being primarily dependent upon somatic mutation or some genetically equivalent process. Since about 1967 most immunologists have accepted the clonal selection approach as a basis for interpreting the production of antibody and with appropriate elaboration the other aspects of the immune response. At the very least all immunological aspects of auto-immune diseases must be discussed within the same framework as normal immune reactions. It is equally logical that the pathological qualities superimposed on the specific reactivity of the immunocytes concerned in auto-immune disease should have a similar origin.

The over-all evidence, including especially the stochastic studies of age and sex incidence by Burch, is consistent with the view that all well-defined auto-immune diseases are based on the occurrence of somatic mutation in a limited number of individual cells. All pathological processes take place in an individual of a certain age and sex with his own genetic make-up and exposed to the normal and exceptional impacts of the environment, including infection, cold, trauma, and the ingestion of drugs. Any of these can, in principle, influence auto-immune processes either by changing the rate at which mutations can emerge into functional visibility or by influencing the activity and effects of the pathogenic clones or their products. Examples of such ancillary aspects of auto-immune disease have been given in many parts of this book.

A brief, final summary of the status of infection, especially slow virus infection, as a 'cause' of auto-immune disease may be helpful in filling out what has already been said in other contexts. In the last analysis, every mutation must have a 'cause', which may be thermal agitation, local ionization, intrusion of reactive alien molecules, or some minor influence of viral or micro-organismal activity (Burnet, 1971). This will hold as much for the somatic mutations that initiate auto-immune clones as for those concerned with malignant change. The type of mutation induced will, however, be completely random in relation to informational content, and, once it has occurred, the subsequent history of the clone will be virtually uninfluenced by the nature of the initiating process.

As will have been evident to any receptive reader, 'auto-immune disease' covers an almost unlimited range of conditions which can only be sorted into nosological entities by some arbitrary decision, for example, that any individual with a consistently positive LE cell test is suffering from SLE or that a patient with rheumatoid arthritis who has swollen parotid glands or dry eyes is a case of Sjögren's syndrome. The whole pattern of heterogeneity, both of clinical course and of pathological and serological findings, is quite unintelligible without the sort of background of germinal and somatic genetic anomalies arising randomly and being chosen for proliferation and survival within the complex adaptive and homoeostatically controlled internal micro-environments of the body.

Epilogue

There is probably a greater total sum of human pain and disability from rheumatoid arthritis, osteo-arthrosis, and related complaints than arises from any other cause. Most of the other conditions we have been concerned with are rarer, but taken together they too add up to a significant sum of human misery. Skilful treatment of the symptoms and disabilities can often comfort the patient and counteract his disabilities, but at a price expressible both in money and in iatrogenic disease. There is at the present time not even a promise of any treatment that can be directed toward the real basis of the auto-immune diseases. It is not in the nature of the medical profession, the drug manufacturers, or the biomedical research community to adopt a pessimistic attitude toward any medical problem. No one is happy when I point out that in the last forty years infectious disease and nutritional disease have been virtually eliminated and treatment and rehabilitation of war injuries and other trauma brought to a remarkable level of effectiveness, but that there has been no basic improvement in the treatment of cancer or auto-immune disease, that the premature death-rate from cardiovascular disease is rising and that much of our extension of life in old age is occupied by the period that someone has appropriately called 'pre-death'.

Auto-immune disease can be a depressing subject. In Shakespearian terms, 'It is a tale told by an idiot, . . . Signifying nothing.' In more modern metaphor, it is an error made at random in an enormous, delicately programmed computer. Depending on the site and nature of the initial error, its result can be trivial or can compound the initial fault into a series of consequences that will make the machine's whole output meaningless. There are many differences between a computer and a man and not all the advantages are on the side of the man. The computer is constructed by engineers and logicians with circuits which can detect and locate errors and allow any faulty component to be removed and replaced by a new one. The mammal, mouse or man, has been constructed by evolution, using a different method of dealing with error: to produce individuals far in excess of the numbers needed and to ensure that those which were functionally less effective were amongst the great majority killed by the impact of the environment before they could reproduce. Nature has no other way of handling genetic error than by eliminating the faulty, and the physician handling auto-immune disease can expect no help from her.

As in all real human problems, there is no solution that can be satisfactory even in principle. We can neither prevent nor cure auto-immune disease. It is an inevitable consequence of the process of organic evolution and the biological necessity for natural death. Like so much else, we can only deal with symptoms as they arise and make an empirical compromise between the needs of the afflicted individuals and the resources of the community.

Abbreviations

ACH	active chronic hepatitis
AD	antigenic determinant
AE	auto-immune encephalitis
AH	auto-immune haemolytic anaemia
AICF	auto-immune complement fixation (test)
ANF	anti-nuclear factor
ARC	antigen-reactive cell
B-	(cell) of the antibody-producing series
CDL	chronic discoid lupus
CL	cardiolipin
CNS	central nervous system
DC	direct Coombs (test)
DH	delayed hypersensitivity
D–L	Donath–Landsteiner
DNP	dinitrophenyl
DPC	dendritic phagocytic cell
EB	Epstein–Barr (virus)
FCA	Freund's complete adjuvant
GALT	gut-associated lymphoid tissue
H	hapten or heavy chain component of antibody, depending on context
HSA	human serum albumin
Ig	immunoglobulin
ITP	idiopathic thrombocytopenic purpura
L	light chain component of antibody
LATS	long-acting thyroid stimulator
LCM	lymphocytic choriomeningitis
LD	lethal dose
LE(cell)	lupus erythematosus
LT	lymphotoxin
MG	myasthenia gravis

MIF	migration inhibitory factor
NZB	New Zealand Black (mice)
PBC	primary biliary cirrhosis
PFC	plaque-forming cell
PHA	phytohaemagglutinin
RF	rheumatoid factor
SLE	systemic lupus erythematosus
T-	thymus-dependent (cells)
TSH	thyroid stimulating hormone
WR	Wassermann reaction

Glossary

It may be helpful to any readers not in touch with recent immunological writing to provide a short list of technical words or phrases commonly used. Most are defined either directly or by implication when first used in the book, but an accessible reminder is often useful.

Agammaglobulinaemia. A condition associated with absence of plasma cells, failure to produce antibody, and very low levels of immunoglobulin in the circulating plasma. There are congenital and acquired forms.

Antibody. An immunoglobulin capable of uniting specifically, by a defined part of its molecule (combining site), with a certain antigenic determinant.

Antigen. Any substance capable of reacting specifically with antibody. Most antigens also stimulate the production of antibody, but when this function is being specifically referred to it is usual to refer to 'immunogen'.

Antigenic determinant. The relatively small chemical configuration which can unite specifically with the combining site of an antibody. There are antigens, such as polymer flagellin, with many identical antigenic determinants, others which carry several qualitatively distinct antigenic determinants.

B-immune system. The system of stem cells, lymphocytes, and plasma cells concerned with the production and liberation of immunoglobulins and antibodies. B derives from the bursa of Fabricius in the chicken, an organ actively associated with the production of such cells. B-cells or B-immunocytes have similar significance.

Blast. A general term for an actively multiplying cell ancestral to specialized cells, as in lymphoblast, plasmablast, fibroblast.

Blastocyst. An early stage of embryonic development with a few dozen cells arranged spherically with some internal fluid.

Clonal selection theory. This holds that the immune pattern of antibody or immunocyte-receptor is determined by genetic processes and that antigen *selects* those immunocytes for proliferation with whose receptors it can unite specifically.

Clone. A population of cells derived from the asexual proliferation of a single parental cell. By convention, when a cell of a clone undergoes somatic mutation or other inheritable change, its descendants constitute a new clone.

Complement. A complex system of proteins in mammalian blood which unites with a variety of antigen–antibody complexes and is usually measured by its power to dissolve (lyse) red blood cells treated with antibody.

Complement-fixation. A serological test system used to detect a specific antibody by allowing it to react with antigen and adding complement. If antibody is present, complement is fixed to the antigen–antibody complex and is unable to lyse 'sensitized' sheep red cells.

Coombs test or antiglobulin test. A means of recognizing that red cells are coated with an immunoglobulin (see p. 121).

Delayed hypersensitivity. A type of reaction seen in an individual who has been 'sensitized' by previous experience of an antigen. In response to an injection, usually intradermal, of a small amount of antigen, an inflamed area appears with a characteristic delay of 12–48 hours.

Fluorescent antibody. Antibody to which fluorescein or some other fluorescent dye has been chemically united. Any site where mutual precipitation of this antibody and its corresponding antigen takes place shows bright fluorescence with ultra-violet illumination.

Freund's complete adjuvant. Used to enhance antibody production and other immune responses. The antigen is given with a mixture of mineral oil and killed tubercle bacilli dispersed as a fine emulsion in saline by the use of a suitable emulsifying agent.

Genome. A general term for the genetic mechanism or the store of genetic information in an organism or an individual cell.

Germinal centres. Regions in lymphoid tissue where proliferation of lymphoblasts is occurring; they are usually regarded as part of the B-immune system.

Hapten. Any substance of relatively low molecular weight which can react as antigenic determinant with antibody but can only act as immunogen (i.e. induce the formation of antibody) when combined with a carrier protein.

Histocompatibility antigens. The set of antigens in tissue cells which determine the rejection response when the tissue is grafted on a genetically distinct animal of the same species.

Immunocyte. Used for any cell which can be shown capable of producing antibody or reacting specifically with an antigen.

Immunoglobulins. Antibodies regarded from the point of view of their structure as proteins (see pp. 33 ff.).

Immunological surveillance. The function, postulated by the author and others, as responsible for the recognition and removal of potentially malignant or other mutant cells in the body.

Karyotype. The number and form of the chromosomes as seen at metaphase in a dividing somatic cell.

Leproma. A swelling of inflammatory tissue seen in one type of leprosy.

Lymphokines. Substances liberated from stimulated lymphocytes which can influence vascular and cellular activity in the local region.

Memory cells. Immunocytes (lymphocytes) whose presence in the body is responsible for the rapid secondary response to an antigen which the individual has previously experienced.

Monoclonal. Indicating that the population of cells concerned has been derived from a single initiating cell.

Mutation. An inheritable change occurring in the DNA of the genome and manifesting itself phenotypically, in descendant organisms or cells, by some functional change. Mutation can occur in somatic cells, such as lymphocytes (somatic mutation), as well as in the germ line.

Myelomatosis. Multiple tumours in the bone marrow associated with proliferation of a malignant plasma cell clone and the appearance of myeloma protein (immunoglobulin) in the blood plasma.

Phenotypic restriction. Most somatic cells and particularly immunocytes carry genetic information which would allow almost any function to be expressed in more than one way. Phenotypic restriction confines expression to only one of the alternatives—one immunocyte, one antibody.

Phytohaemagglutinin (PHA). A kidney bean extract agglutinating red cells and stimulating lymphocytes to blast transformation and mitosis.

Pure line strains. Strains of experimental animals, commonly mice, which, as a result of close inbreeding, are made up of individuals that are genetically uniform. The following terms are used in discussing transplantation experiments: *syngeneic*, when graft tissues are from the same strain as the recipient; *allogeneic*, from an individual of a different strain of the same species; *xenogeneic*, from a different species.

Stochastic. Referring to the type of logical and mathematical treatment applicable to the regularities that arise when large numbers of random events are recorded.

Thymectomy. Surgical removal of the thymus; neonatal thymectomy: when done within 24 hours from birth.

T-immune system. Immunocytes and their progenitor cells which, before becoming functionally active, require either to multiply within the thymus or be influenced by a thymic hormone. T-immunocytes do not liberate antibody and are responsible for delayed hypersensitivity, rejection of foreign tissues, and other functions.

Tolerance or immunological unresponsiveness. A condition in which an animal fails to produce an immune response when exposed to injections or other manipulations that in other animals would regularly be effective.

References

No attempt has been made to provide references for every significant statement, but the following list, by chapters, includes all the references specifically quoted in the text and a selection of reviews, texts, or key papers which have been consulted and may be useful to the reader.

Chapter 1

General: The approach used derives from my own development of clonal selection theory in:

The Clonal Selection Theory of Acquired Immunity, Vanderbilt and Cambridge University Presses (1959).

Cellular Immunology, Melbourne and Cambridge University Presses (1969).

Basic information on auto-immunity and auto-immune disease has come largely from:

Recent volumes of *Advances in Immunology*.

Clinical Aspects of Immunology, ed. P. G. N. Gell and R. R. A. Coombs, 2nd edition. Blackwell, Oxford (1968).

Immunological Diseases, ed. M. Samter and H. L. Alexander. Little, Brown, Boston (1965).

Autoimmune Diseases, I. R. Mackay and F. M. Burnet. Thomas, Springfield, Illinois (1963).

Chapter 2

References to most of Burch's papers will be found in his book:

BURCH, P. R. J. *An Inquiry Concerning Growth, Disease and Ageing*. Oliver and Boyd, Edinburgh (1968).

The graphs in Fig. 6 are from

BURCH, P. R. J., and ROWELL, N. R., 'Autoimmunity: Aetiological aspects of chronic discoid and systemic lupus erthyematosis, systemic sclerosis, and Hashimoto's thyroiditis', *Lancet*, **ii**, 507 (1963).

BURCH, P. R. J., and ROWELL, N. R. 'Lupus erythematosus', *Acta derm.-venereol.* (*Stockholm*), **50**, 293 (1970).

BULLOUGH, W. S. 'Ageing of mammals', *Nature*, **229**, 608 (1971).

FISHER, B., SZUCH, P., LEVINE, M., and FISHER, E. R. 'A portal blood factor as the humoral agent in liver regeneration', *Science*, **171**, 575 (1971).

FRASER, A. S., and SHORT, B. F. 'Studies of sheep mosaic for fleece type. I. Patterns and origins of mosaicism', *Austr. J. biol. Sciences*, **11**, 200 (1958).

KNUDSON, A. C. 'Mutation and cancer: statistical study of retinoblastoma', *Proc. nat. Acad. Sci. Wash.* **68**, 820 (1971).

Chapter 3

BOYSE, E. A. 'Organization and modulation of cell membrane receptors', in *Immunologic Surveillance*, ed. R. T. Smith and M. Landy, p. 5. Academic Press, New York and London (1970).

MILLER, J. F. A. P., BASTEN, A., SPRENT, J., and CHEERS C. 'Interaction between lymphocytes in immune response', *Cellular Immunology*, **2**, 469 (1971).

WANG, A. C., WILSON, S. K., HOPPER, J. E., FUDENBERG, H. H., and NISONOFF, A. 'Evidence for control of synthesis of the variable regions of the heavy chains of immunoglobulins G and M by the same gene', *Proc. nat. Acad. Sci. Wash.* **66**, 337 (1970).

Chapter 4

DRESSER, D. W., and MITCHISON, N. A. 'The mechanism of immunological paralysis', *Advances in Immunology*, **8**, 129, ed. F. J. Dixon and H. G. Kunkel. Academic Press, New York and London (1968).

HUMPHREY, J. H. 'Immunological unresponsiveness to protein antigens in rabbits. I. The duration of unresponsiveness following a single injection at birth. II. The nature of the subsequent antibody response', *Immunology*, **7**, 449 and 462 (1964).

NOSSAL, G. J. V., and ADA, C. L. *Antigens, Lymphoid Cells and the Immune Response.* Academic Press, New York and London (1971).

PARISH, C. R. 'Immune response to chemically modified flagellin. I. Induction of antibody tolerance to flagellin by aceto-acetylated derivatives of the protein. II. Evidence for a fundamental relationship between humoral and cell-mediated immunity', *J. exp. Med.* **134**, 1 and 21 (1971).

Chapter 5

McFarland, W. 'Microspikes on the lymphocyte uropod', *Science*, **163**, 818 (1969).
Miledi, R., Molinoff, P., and Potter, L. T. 'Isolation of the cholinergic receptor protein of *Torpedo* electric tissue', *Nature*, **229**, 554 (1971).
Nossal, G. J. V., and Ada, C. L. *Antigens, Lymphoid Cells and the Immune Response*. Academic Press, New York and London (1971).
Paton, W. D. M. 'Receptors as defined by their pharmacological properties', in *Molecular Properties of Drug Receptors*, ed. R. Porter and M. O'Connor, p. 3. CIBA Foundation Symposium. Churchill, London (1970).

Chapter 6

Burnet, F. M. *Cellular Immunology*. Melbourne and Cambridge University Presses (1969).
Wright, D. J. M., Doniach, D., Lessof, M. H., Turk, J. L., Grimble, A. S., and Catterall, R. D. 'New antibody in early syphilis', *Lancet*, **i**, 740 (1970).

Chapter 7

Elkins, W. L. 'The interaction of donor and host lymphoid cells in the pathogenesis of renal cortical destruction induced by a local graft versus host reaction', *J. exp. Med.* **123**, 103 (1966).
Rose, N. R. Metzgar, R. S., and Witebsky, E. 'Studies on organ specificity. XI. Isoantigens of rabbit pancreas', *J. Immunol.* **85**, 575 (1960).
Steiner, J. W., Langer, B., Schatz, D. L., and Volpe, R. 'Experimental immunologic adrenal injury: a response to injections of autologous and homologous adrenal antigens in adjuvant', *J. exp. Med.* **112**, 187 (1960).

Chapter 8

In this chapter, which I regard as of special importance to the discussion, I have deviated from the rule that holds for all other chapters and included a considerable number of recent references. The approach adopted has not previously been published and it seemed desirable to give the main relevant references.

General review

HOWIE, J. B., and HELYER, B. J. 'The immunology and pathology of NZB mice', in *Advances in Immunology*, **9**, 215, ed. F. J. Dixon and H. G. Kunkel. Academic Press, New York and London (1968).

ALLMAN, V., GHAFFAR, A., PLAYFAIR, J. H. L., and ROITT, I. M. 'Transfer of autoantibody formation by NZB bone marrow cells', *Transplantation*, **8**, 899 (1969).

BIELSCHOWSKY, M., and GOODALL, C. M. 'Origin of inbred NZ mouse strains', *Cancer Res.* **30**, 834 (1970).

HOLBOROW, E. J., BARNES, R. D. S., and TUFFREY, M. 'A new red-cell autoantibody in NZB mice', *Nature*, **207**, 601 (1965).

HOLMES, M. C., and BURNET, F. M. 'The inheritance of auto-immune disease in mice: a study of hybrids of the strains NZB and C3H', *Heredity*, **19**, 419 (1964).

HOLMES, M. C., GORRIE, J., and BURNET, F. M. 'Transmission by splenic cells of an autoimmune disease occurring spontaneously in mice', *Lancet*, **ii**, 638 (1961).

KAYE, D., and HOOK, E. W. 'Influence of autoimmune hemolytic anemia on susceptibility to *Salmonella* infection', *Proc. Soc. exp. Biol. Med.* **117**, 20 (1964).

LINDSEY, E. S., and WOODRUFF, M. F. A. 'The effect of irradiation and infusion of marrow and spleen cells on autoimmune anaemia in NZB/B1 mice', *Proc. R. Soc. Med.* **60**, 826 (1967).

MASON, S., and WARNER, N. 'Analysis of plasma cell tumour "mutants"', *Walter and Eliza Hall Institute Annual Report*, p. 50 (1969/70).

MORTON, J. I., and SIEGEL, B. V. 'Response of NZB mice to foreign antigen and development of autoimmune disease,' *J. reticuloendothel. Soc.* **6**, 78 (1969).

NORINS, L. C., and HOLMES, M. C. 'Antinuclear factor in mice', *J. Immunol.* **93**, 148 (1964).

RUSSELL, P. J., HICKS, J. D., BOSTON, L. E., and ABBOTT, A. 'Failure to transfer haemolytic anaemia or glomerulonephritis with cell-free material from NZB mice', *Clin. exp. Immunol.* **6**, 227 (1970).

STAPLES, P. J., and TALAL, N. 'Rapid loss of tolerance induced in weanling NZB and B/W F1 mice', *Science*, **163**, 1215 (1969).

STEINBERG, A. D., BARON, S., and TALAL, N. 'The pathogenesis of autoimmunity in New Zealand mice. I. Induction of antinucleic acid antibodies by polyinosinic-polycytidylic acid', *Proc. nat. Acad. Sci. Wash.* **63**, 1102 (1969).

WARNER, N. L., and MOORE, M. A. S. 'Defects in hematopoietic differentiation in NZB and NZC mice', *J. exp. Med.* **134**, 313 (1971).

WILSON, J. D., WARNER, N. L., and HOLMES, M. C. 'Autoantibody-secreting plaque forming cells in spleen and thymus of NZB and normal mice', *Nature new Biol.*, **233**, 80 (1971).

Chapter 9

For a review of AHA:

DACIE, J. V. *The Haemolytic Anaemias: Congenital and Acquired*, Part 2, 2nd edition. Churchill, London (1962).

BURNET, F. M. 'Immunological surveillance in neoplasia', *Transplantation Reviews*, **7**, 3 (1971).

LEDDY, J. P., and BAKEMEIER, R. F. 'Structural aspects of human erythrocyte autoantibodies. I. L chain types and electrophoretic dispersion,' *J. exp. Med.* **121**, 1 (1965).

SHULMAN, N. R., MARDER, V. J., and WEINRACH, R. S. 'Similarities between known antiplatelet antibodies and the factor responsible for thrombocytopenia in idiopathic purpura. Physiologic, serologic and isotopic studies', *Ann. N.Y. Acad. Sci.* **124**, 499 (1965).

SHULMAN, N. R., and HIRSCHMAN, R. J. 'Acquired hemophilia', *Trans. Ass. Amer. Physicians*, **82**, 388 (1969).

Chapter 10

General clinical review:

BOYLE, J. A., and BUCHANAN, W. W. *Clinical Rheumatology*. Blackwell, Oxford (1971).

BURCH, P. R. J. *An Inquiry Concerning Growth, Disease and Ageing*. Oliver and Boyd, Edinburgh (1968).

BURCH, P. R. J., and ROWELL, N. R. 'Lupus erthyematosus', *Acta derm.-vener. (Stockholm)*, **50**, 293 (1970).
TALAL, N. 'Sjögren's syndrome, lymphoproliferation, and renal tubular acidosis', *Ann. intern. Med.* **74**, 633 (1971).

Chapter 11

BAUR, S., FISHER, J. M., STRICKLAND, R. G., and TAYLOR, K. B. 'Autoantibody-containing cells in the gastric mucosa in pernicious anaemia', *Lancet*, **ii**, 887 (1968).
DONIACH, D., ROITT, I. M., and TAYLOR, K. B. 'Autoimmunity in pernicious anaemia and thyroiditis: a family study', *Ann. N.Y. Acad. Sci.* **124**, 605 (1965).
GOLDSTEIN, G., and MACKAY, I. R. *The Human Thymus.* Heinemann Medical Books, London (1969).
GOLDSTEIN, G., and WHITTINGHAM, S. 'Experimental autoimmune thymitis: an animal model of human myasthenia gravis', *Lancet*, **ii**, 315 (1966).
HOFFMANN, M. J., HETZEL, B. S., and MANSON, J. 'Neonatal thyrotoxicosis: report of three cases involving four infants', *Austr. Ann. Med.*, **15**, 262 (1966).
KNOWLES, M., SAUNDERS, M., CURRIE, S., WALTON, J. N., and FIELD, E. J. 'Lymphocyte transformation in the Guillain-Barré syndrome', *Lancet*, **ii**, 1168 (1969).
PIERPAOLI, W., BARONI, C., FABRIS, N., and SORKIN, E. 'Hormones and immunological capacity. II. Reconstitution of antibody production in hormonally deficient mice by somatotropic hormone, thyrotropic hormone and thyroxin', *Immunology*, **16**, 217 (1969).
VETTERS, J. M., SIMPSON, J. A., and FOLKARDE, A. 'Experimental myasthenia gravis', *Lancet*, **ii**, 28 (1969).

Chapter 12

BURNET, F. M. *Immunological Surveillance.* Pergamon Press Australia, Sydney (1970).
COSTEA, N., YAKULIS, V. J., and HELLER, P. 'The mechanism of induction of cold agglutinins by mycoplasma pneumoniae', *J. Immunol.* **106**, 598 (1971).
KAHN, M. F., RYCKEWAERT, A., CANNAT, A., SOLNICA, J., and DE SEZE, S. 'Systemic lupus erythematosus and ovarian dys-

germinoma: remission of the SLE after extirpation of the tumour', *Clin. exp. Immunol.* **1**, 355 (1966).

Chapter 13

COLLIER, H. O. J. 'Prostaglandins and aspirin', *Nature*, **232**, 17 (1971).

BURNET, F. M. *The Background of Infectious Diseases in Man.* Melbourne Postgraduate Committee, Melbourne (1946).

Chapter 14

For general discussions of ageing see:

BURNET, F. M. 'An immunological approach to ageing', *Lancet*, **ii**, 358 (1970).

COMFORT, A. *Ageing: The Biology of Senescence*, 2nd edition. Holt, Rinehart and Winston, New York (1964).

WALFORD, R. L. *The Immunologic Theory of Aging.* Munksgaard, Copenhagen (1969).

HAYFLICK, L. 'The limited *in vitro* lifetime of human diploid cell strains', *Exp. Cell Res.* **37**, 614 (1965).

JONES, H. B. 'The relation of human health to age, place and time', in *Handbook of Ageing and the Individual*, ed. J. E. Birren. University of Chicago Press (1959).

Chapter 15

DIENER, E., and ARMSTRONG, W. D. 'Immunological tolerance *in vitro*: kinetic studies at the cellular level', *J. exp. Med.* **129**, 591 (1969).

Index

Acquired tolerance, 68
  see also Immunological tolerance
Acromegaly, see Auto-immune diseases
Agammaglobulinaemia, 48–9, 53, 54, 88, 214
  see also Auto-immune diseases
Ageing: biology of, 201–3
  see also Auto-immune disease: age incidence
Aleutian mink disease, 92–3
Amyloid disease, 48
Ankylosing spondytis, see Rheumatoid arthritis: age incidence of
Antibodies, 33–43, 48, 53–7, 101
  anti-tumour, 54
  D-L antibody, 125–6
  genetic determination of, 38
  production of, 33–4, 37, 39, 50–1, 53, 55, 61, 63, 69, 75, see also Antigens
  see also Immunoglobulin and specific diseases, e.g. Systemic lupus erythematosus
Antibody diversity, 39–43
Antigen-antibody complexes, 83, 187–9
  investigation of using bovine serum albumin, 82
Antigen-antibody reactions, 69, 73
Antigen-immunocyte reactions, 73, 76–7
Antigen-receptor interactions, 65–6, 68
Antigenic determinants, 33–7, 40–1, 54, 60, 64–6, 67, 69, 81, 97, 102, 173
  collagen, 69, 211–12
  dinitrophenyl group, 42
  elastin, 69
  self antigenic determinants, 64
  see also Haptens, Anti-haptens
Antigens, 37, 39, 43, 46, 49–50, 54, 64, 98
  artificial, 69
  ectopic production of by tumours, 186–7
  specific tissue, 99–101
  specificity of, 46, 54
  stimulation of immunocyte (ARC), 74–7
  synthetic peptide, 39
  see also Antibodies: production of
Anti-haptens, 92
  see also Antigenic determinants, Haptens
Anti-immunoglobulins, 139
Anti-inflammatory drugs, 194
Antimalarials: treatment of auto-immune disease, 194
Astrocytes: immunological functions of, 96
Ataxia-telangiectasia, 94
Auto-antibodies, 54, 65, 91–2, 97–8, 104, 118, 213
  hapten-carrier hypothesis, 99–101
Auto-antigens, 196–8
  see also DNA
Auto-immune disease, 2–8, 9, 25, 41, 48, 54–6, 59, 65–71, 80, 82, 85, 91–7, 118, 121, 131–51
  age incidence of, 6–7, 18–25, 201–12
  drug therapy of, 192–8
  graft-versus-host reaction, 104–7
  laboratory investigations of, 216–18
  localized, 98, 103–4, 153–71, 174
  pathogenesis of, 173–90
  population genetics of, 214–15
  prevention of, 191
  sex incidence of, 18
  simulation in normal animals, 97
  specific organs, 182–6
  surgical treatment of, 194–6

Auto-immune disease—*cont.*
  therapy of, 191–9, *see also* names of drugs and diseases
Auto-immune diseases
  acromegaly, 153
  adrenals, 81–2, 104, 182
  encephalonyelitis, 81–2, 83, 98, 101–3
  haemolytic anaemia, 84, 92–3, 105, 109, 110, 121–6, 132, 178–82, 184
    cold type, 124–6
    drug induced, 182, 191
    drug therapy of, 191
    surgical treatment of, 195
    warm type, 123–4, 216
  haemophilia, 129
  Hashimoto's disease, 82, 101, 154–8, 160, 166, 185
  hyperthyroidism, 153
  idiopathic Addison's disease, 153, 162–3
  iodiopathic thrombocytopenic purpura, 127–9
    surgical treatment of, 195
  liver, 163–5
  myasthenia gravis, 153, 165–7
    surgical treatment of, 195
  nervous system, 170
  neuritis, 81
    of the blood, 154–61, 166, 182
  thyroid, 154–61, 166, 182
    pathogenesis of, 158–60
  see also NZB mice, specific diseases, e.g. systemic lupus erythematosus
Auto-immune response, *see* Immune response
Auto-immunity, 2–8, 25, 47, 53, 56, 69
Auto-immunocytes, 75, 84, 97
Azathioprine: treatment of auto-immune diseases, 192, 196, 199, 207

B-chains, 34–6, 48–51, 54–5, 60
B-immunocytes, 62, 64, 68–9, 75, 77, 88, 89–90, 91–2, 99–100, 103–4, 127, 160, 161–2
Birthmarks, 14–15
B-lymphocytes, 60
Blood cells
  diseases of, 121–9
  see also Auto-immune diseases, Leukopenias, Pancytopenias
Bone marrow, 49, 66, 113, 128
  generation of stem cells, 45, 98
  tumours in, 48
Bursa of Fabricus, 43, 49
  ageing of, 204–5

Cancer, 3, 14, 20
  see also specific diseases, e.g. Retinoblastoma
Cell proliferation
  limits to, 203–6
Cells
  antibody producing, 65
  antigen reactive, 32
  differentiation of, 37–8, 43
  differentiation to immunocytes, 43–5
  growth of, 26–32, *see also* Mitosis
  infiltration of, 80–2
  mutation of, 37
  plaque forming, 55, 114–15, 117, 128
  population dynamics of, 28–9, 32, 43–5
  population genetics of, 28–32
  somatic mutation of, 47, 117, 202, 204, 209–12
Cellular immunology, 31
Chalone theory, 26–7
Chimera, 60
Chloroquine: treatment of auto-immune disease, 194
Chronic discoid lupus: age incidence of, 24–5
Clonal selection theory, 2–4, 9
  see also Forbidden clones
Clones
  auto-immune, 43, 70, 82
  IgG producing, 37
  IgM producing, 37
  see also Forbidden clones: Myeloma clone
Cloning of immunocytes, 216–18
Collagen, *see* Antigenic determinants: collagen
Coombs test, 105, 110–13, 114, 121–2, 178–80, 217

Cortico-steroids: treatment of auto-immune diseases, 192, 193–4, 199
Cortisol: treatment of auto-immune diseases, 193
Cortisone: treatment of auto-immune disease, 193
Creuzfeldt-Jakob disease, 94, 170
Cushings syndrome, 159–60, 168
  induced by drugs, 194
Cyclophosphamide: treatment of auto-immune disease, 192, 196
Cytotoxic drugs: treatment of auto-immune disease, 191, 192, 196

Delayed-hypersensitivity, 51–2, 62, 70
Dendritic phagocytic cells, 63
Dermatomyositis, 148–51, 186
Determinant: antigenic, *see* Antigenic determinants
Diabetes insipidus, 159–60
Dinitrophenyl group, *see* Antigenic determinants: dinitrophenyl group
DNA: auto-antigen in systemic lupus erythematosus, 133
Drug receptors, 73–4
Drug therapy, *see* Auto-immune disease: drug therapy
Dysgammaglobulinaemia, 47

Elastin, *see* Antigenic determinants: elastin
Encephalitogenic protein, 98
Eosinophils, 80
Erosive arthritis, *see* Rheumatoid arthritis: age incidence of

Felty syndrome, *see* Rheumatoid arthritis: variants of
Forbidden clones, 3–9, 18–22, 97, 107, 111, 126, 141, 173–90, 195–6, 214
Freckles, 11–13
Freund's complete adjuvant, 97–9, 103–4, 154, 183

Gammaglobulin, 68
Gastric atrophy, 160–1
  see also Auto-immune diseases
Genes: intragenomic interaction between, 38
Gold compounds: treatment of auto-immune disease, 194
Graft-versus-host reaction, 97, 183
  model of auto-immune disease, 104–7
  see also Auto-immune disease: graft-versus-host reaction
Grave's disease, 156–7, 158, 160
  surgical treatment of, 195
Guillain-Barré syndrome, 170

Haemoglobinuria, 125
Haemolytic anaemia, *see* Auto-immune diseases: haemolytic anaemia
Haemophilia, *see* Auto-immune diseases: haemophilia
Haptens, 33, 41, 51, 61
  cardiolipin, 92
  phospholipid, 91
  see also Anti-haptens, Antigenic-determinants
Hashimoto's disease, *see* Auto-immune diseases: Hashimoto's disease
Hepatitis, 132, 191, 192, 199
  see also Auto-immune disease
High-zone tolerance, 70, 75
Hodgkin's disease, 47
Homologous disease, *see* Graft-versus-host reaction
Human serum albumin: injection into rabbits, 67
  annihilation of immunocytes, 68
Hydralazine, *see* Systemic lupus erythematosus: drug induced
Hyperthyroidism, *see* Auto-immune diseases: hyperthyroidism

Iatrogenic disease, 199
Idiopathic Addison's disease, *see* Auto-immune diseases: idiopathic Addison's disease
Idiopathic thrombocytopenic purpura, *see* Auto-immune diseases: idiopathic thrombocytopenic purpura

Immune competance, 67
Immune response, 62–3, 67
B-system, 88–9, 90–2, 99–104, 128, 160–2
haemolytic anaemia, 123–4
normal animals, 97–105
NZB mice, 115–16
pharmacological aspects, 73–85
T-system, 64, 88–9, 90–2, 94–5, 98, 99–104, 128, 134, 139, 160–2, 174, 213
viral disease, 87–9
Immunity, 48–51, 56
B-system, 48–55, 60
cellular aspects of, 73–85
diversity of immune patterns, 36–43
T-system, 48–55, 60
Immunocytes, 32–3, 37–8, 40–5, 47, 49, 54, 64, 73, 81
annihilation by HSA, 68
cell cultures of, 84
population dynamics of, 43–5
see also Auto-immunocytes
Immunoglobulin chains, 34–7
amino-acid sequences of, 35
Immunoglobulin receptors, 43
Immunoglobulins, 30–2, 33–7, 41, 43, 44, 46, 47
Ig A, 33, 35–7, 43, 44, 47, 55, 62
Ig D, 33, 35–7, 43, 44, 47, 55, 62
Ig E, 33, 35–7, 43, 44, 47, 55, 62
Ig G, 33–7, 43, 44, 47, 48, 50, 55–6, 62, 112–14, 131, 132, 139, 188
Ig M, 33, 35–7, 43, 44, 47, 48, 50, 55, 62, 139, 188
chemical structure, 34–6
immune pattern of, 37
production of, 37
see also Anti-immunoglobulins, Antibodies, Myeloma proteins
Immunological paralysis, 59–71
Immunological surveillance, 206–9
Immunological tolerance, 59–71, 174, 196–8
allophenic mice, 174
NZB mice, 115, 118
rats, 69–70
role of T-immunocytes, 68–71
skin, 60, 100–2, 104
see also Acquired tolerance, Natural tolerance, Partial tolerance
Immunology, 33–57
cellular aspects, 43–5
Immunosuppressive drugs, 196–8, 207
see also specific drugs, e.g. Azathioprine
Indomethacin: treatment of auto-immune disease, 194
Infection, 87–96
slow virus, 92–6
Inflammatory arthritis, *see* Rheumatoid arthritis: age incidence of
Intrinsic tolerance, 63–6

Joint affections, *see* Rheumatoid arthritis: age incidence of

Kidney disease, 131
Kuru, 92–6, 170

Leucocytes, 53, 79
Leukaemia, 47, 123
Leukopenias, 128–9
Liver disease, *see* Auto-immune diseases: liver disease
Localized auto-immune diseases, *see* Auto-immune disease: localized
Low zone tolerance, 70
Lymphoblasts, 30, 61
see also Lymphocytes, Plasmablasts
Lymphocytes, 26, 29–32, 49, 52, 80, 102
circulation of, 80–2
mitosis of, 30
population dynamics of, 45–8
production of lymphokines, 78
resistance of lympotoxins, 79
transformation to Kupfer cells, 43
see also Lymphoblasts, Plasmablasts, Thymocytes
Lymphocytic choriomeningitis: mice 87–8
Lymphocytic leukaemia, 123
Lymphoid tissue: tumours of, 94
Lymphokines, 50–2, 64, 77–9, 194
Lymphoma, 123
Lymphosarcoma, 47

Macroglobulinaemia, 145
Macrophages, 43, 53, 63
Mast cells, 44, 80, 204
  production of histamine, 79
  role in immune responses, 79–80
Measles: immune response to, 88
Melanocytes, 10–16
  α-methyldopa: treatment of auto-immune disease, 198
Mitosis, 26–7, 204
  inhibitors, 26–7
  stimulators, 27
Mitotic control proteins, 26– 7
Monoclonal dysgammaglobulinaemia, 47
Monocytes, 52, 80, 102
Multiple myeloma, 46–8, 217
  NZB mice, 115
Multiple sclerosis, 170
Myasthenia gravis, *see* Auto-immune diseases: myasthenia gravis
Myeloma clone, 47
Myeloma proteins, 37, 41, 46–8, 207
Myelomatosis, *see* Multiple myeloma

Natural tolerance, 59–62
  see also Immunological tolerance
Nervous system: diseases of, *see* Auto-immune diseases: nervous sytem
Neuritis, *see* Auto-immune diseases, neuritis
Neuromyopathies, 186
NZB mice, 109–19, 135, 188, 215–16
  auto-immune disease in, 110–11
  future investigations on, 218–19
  genetic factors, 111–13
  haemolytic anaemia in, 110, 117–19, 178–80, 184
  immunological response in, 115–16
  kidney disease, 110
  plaque forming cells, 114–15, 128
  somatic factors, 111–13, 117–19
  transfer of cells from NZB mice to other mice, 113–14
  see also Auto-immune diseases: haemolytic anaemia, immunological response, immunological tolerance, multiple myeloma, virus infection

Ophthalmia, *see* Sympathetic ophthalmia
Osteo-arthritis, 221
  treatment of, 192
  see also Rheumatoid arthritis: age incidence of
Ovarian dysgerminoma, 187

Pancytopenias, 128–9
Partial tolerance, 66–71
  rats, 70
  see also Immunological tolerance
Periarteritis nodosa, 148
Pernicious anaemia, 160–1
  see also Auto-immune disease
Phenotypic restriction, 37–8, 43–5
Phenylbutazone: treatment of auto-immune disease, 194
Phytohaemagglutinin, 50
Plasma cells, 204
  antibody secreting, 46
  mutation of, 37, 44
Plasmablasts, 30, 47
  see also Lymphoblasts, Lymphocytes
Platelets, 127–8
Polyarteritis nodosa, 148–51
Polymyositis, 148
Prednisone: treatment of auto-immune disease, 193
Procainamide, *see* Systemic lupus erythematosus: drug induced
Progressive systemic sclerosis, 148

Radiation: Effect on NZB mice, 114, 115
Raynaud's disease, 125
Renal transplants, 207
Reticulosarcoma, 123
Retinoblastoma, 20–3
Rh antibodies, 121
Rh antigen, 54–5, 123
Rheumatic fever
  genetic predisposition to, 90
  immune response to, 89–91
Rheumatoid arthritis, 25, 132, 138–51, 187–8, 208, 220–1

Rheumatoid arthritis—*cont.*
  age incidence of, 145–7
  antibodies, 139–44
  anti-immunoglobulins, 139–44
  etiology of, 139–44
  genetic factors, 145–7
  immune response in, 142–4
  immune receptor patterns, 142
  prevention of, 191
  somatic mutations, 145–7
  treatment, 194
  variants of, 144–51
Rheumatoid factor, *see* Rheumatoid arthritis
Runt disease, *see* Graft-versus-host reaction

Salmonella flagellar protein: antigen in rats, 69–70, 197, 216
Scrapie, 92–6, 170
Self antigenic determinants, *see* Antigenic determinants: self antigenic determinants
Self antigens, 66
Sjogren's syndrome, 82, 147–8, 220
  see also Rheumatoid arthritis: variants of
Skin
  albinos, 16
  homografts in mice, 68
  moles on, 14–15
  pigmentation, 10–11, 16
  sheep, 16–18
  somatic mutation in, 10–18
  sunburn, 10–13
Slow virus infection, 92–6
Smallpox: immune response to, 89
Snake venom: pharmacological activities of, 74
Splenectomy, 197, 216
Stem cells, 37, 38, 43, 47, 49, 128
  origin of, 45–6, 98
Stibophen, *see* Auto-immune diseases: haemalytic anaemia: drug induced
Still's disease, *see* Rheumatoid arthritis: variants of
Stochastic models, 9–32
Surgery, *see* Auto-immune disease: surgical treatment of
Sympathetic ophthalmia, 171
Synthetic peptide antigens, *see* Antigens: synthetic peptide
Syphilis
  congenital in children, 125
  immune response to, 91–2
  treatment of, 191
Systemic lupus erythematosus, 14, 123, 131–8, 140, 148–9, 151, 164, 185, 187, 188, 190, 210, 214–15, 219–20
  antibodies in, 132–4, 136
  drug induced, 134–5, 138, 198
  genetic influence on, 135–6, 138
  immune response in, 136
  immunopathology, 135–8
  LE-cell test, 131–2, 133, 134
  production of immunocytes, 137
  treatment of, 192–4
Systemic rheumatoid disease, *see* Rheumatoid arthritis: variants of
Systemic sclerosis, 148, 149–51

T-immunocytes, 62, 65, 76–7, 88–95, 98–104, 127, 134, 139, 160–2, 174, 213
  role in tolerance, 68–71
Thrombocytopenic purpura, 126–9, 132, 191
  treatment of, 191
Thymectomy, 195, 216
Thymocytes, 46, 174
Thymomas, 167–9
Thymosin, 46
Thymus, 43–6, 49, 56, 66
  ageing of, 204–5
  liberation of hormones, 44
  mice, 43–6
Thymus-dependent immune responses, 44–6, 165–8
Thymus-independent immune responses, 50–5
Thyroid: diseases of, *see* Auto-immune diseases: thyroid
Thyroidectomy, 195
Thyroiditis: experimentally induced in rabbits, 103–4
Thyrotoxicosis, 210
Tolerance, *see* Immunological tolerance

Tuberculin
  injection into guinea pigs, 78
  Mantoux reaction to, 48
Tumours
  bronchial carcinomas, 186–7
  ectopic production of antigens, 186–7

Virus infection, 87–96, 220
  NZB mice, 111, 116–17
  oncogenic virus, 116–17

Wasserman reaction, 91–2, 100, 133–4

X-irradiation: inducement of autoimmune haemolytic anaemia and thrombocytopenic purpura, 191

GPSR Compliance

The European Union's (EU) General Product Safety Regulation (GPSR) is a set of rules that requires consumer products to be safe and our obligations to ensure this.

If you have any concerns about our products, you can contact us on ProductSafety@springernature.com

In case Publisher is established outside the EU, the EU authorized representative is:

Springer Nature Customer Service Center GmbH
Europaplatz 3
69115 Heidelberg, Germany

Batch number: 10583998

Printed by Printforce, the Netherlands